5:2 Fasting Diet For Beginners

50 Recipes to Detox, Lose Weight and Age Gracefully

By

Sharon Daniels

Legal Disclaimers and Notices

Table of Contents

Part 1: Intermittent Fasting

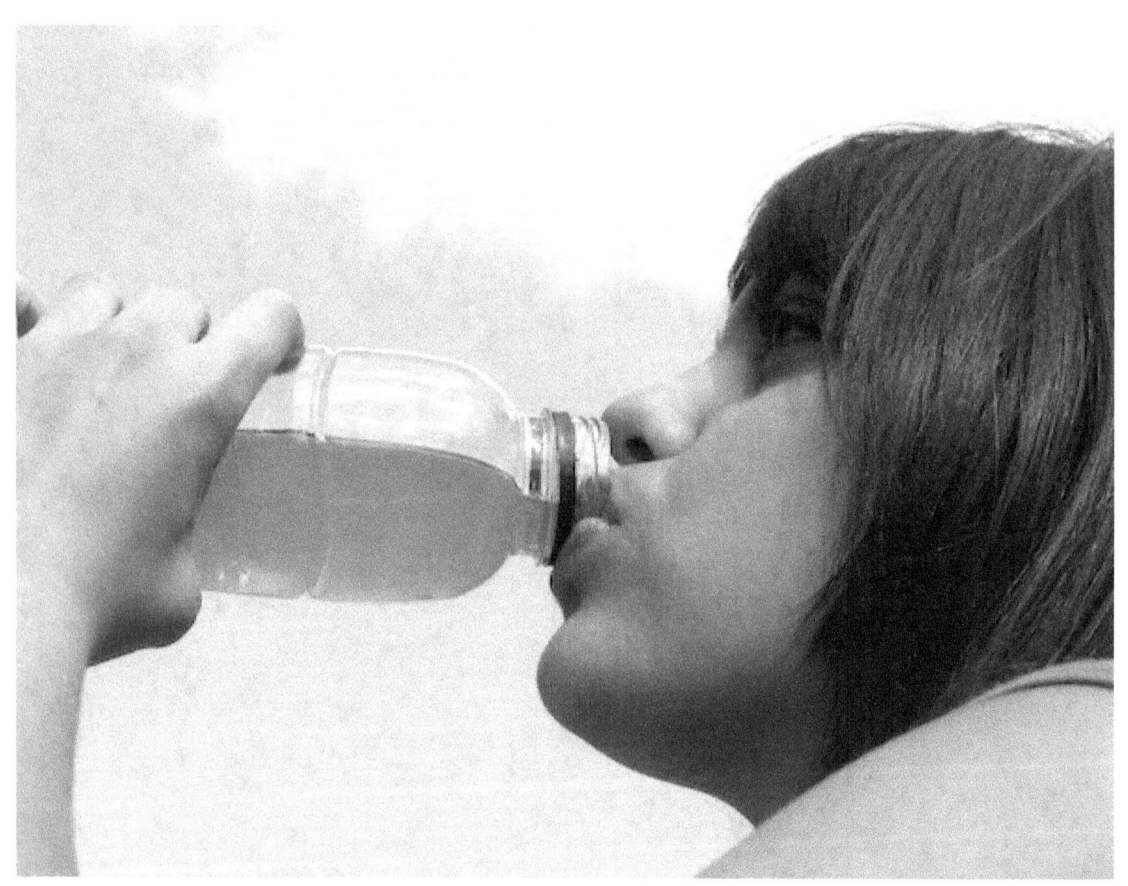

A Look at Intermittent Fasting

For years, using Intermittent Fasting (IF) as a method to lose weight has repeatedly proved to be both simple and efficient. There are no expensive supplements or pre-packaged meals to buy, no points to count, no embarrassing weekly weigh-ins to endure. It is just you - at home, work, or play – eating normally the entire week long while incorporating a small and simple fast mixed in there somewhere. Traditional INTERMITTENT FASTING involves fasting every other day or every third day. However, there are different Intermittent Fasting options available. After about a few months' worth of fasting, people typically find a fast/feed cycle that works best for them.

There are only two major rules to INTERMITTENT FASTING:
1. INTERMITTENT FASTING fasts should last no less than 16 hours and no more than 48 hours at a time.
2. During the fasting duration, you are to consume ONLY water, green tea, or the occasional raw natural fruit juice.

What is Intermittent Fasting (IF)

Intermittent fasting is the ideal way to lose weight without losing muscle mass. As a matter of fact, intermittent fasting does for your body what an intense cardiovascular workout would do. Intermittent fasting involves weekly rotations of feeding and fasting. This helps with weight loss because these cycles keep your body guessing and working hard, which sends your metabolic rate into overdrive and helps maintain a fast metabolism. The more consistent you are with your feeding and fasting, the faster you will reach your weight loss goals.

Take a look at the two most common myths about intermittent fasting:

Myth: Intermittent Fasting will slow down your metabolism.

Many people attempting to lose weight fear fasting will only slow down their metabolism – this is only true for fasting that lasts three or more consecutive days. With intermittent fasting, such as the 5:2 diet, short intervals of fasting (no more than a day or two at a time) will actually speed up your metabolism during the duration of the fast, but because your body does not fall into starvation mode during a two-day fast (you are just tricking your body into thinking it's starving), your metabolism will stay at a speedy, unwavering state during both your fasting and feeding days.

Myth: Intermittent Fasting will lead to muscle loss.

Intermittent fasting does not produce muscle loss. In fact, you will actually perform better, exercise harder, have more energy, and more strength during a fast! Remember – I am speaking of INTERMITTENT fasting only (2 days or less). If you were to fast for more than 3 consecutive days, then you could be at risk for muscle loss and your body would be weakened. Through intermittent fasting, your body is actually capable of producing muscle mass more quickly if you adjust your feeding and fasting days as needed. With intermittent fasting, your body knows no bounds. You will be surprised over how much better you feel – even after just one fast!

Pros and Cons of Intermittent Fasting

As with anything there are pros and cons. What's important is that the pros significantly outweigh the cons and with intermittent fasting, this is absolutely the case. The benefits that are received through intermittent fasting considerably outweigh any risks that may be associated with this lifestyle. Here are some of the more notable pros and cons related to intermittent fasting:

Pros:

➢ Irregular eating cycles can promote insulin and blood sugar balance.

➢ 1- and 2-day fasting reduces body fat while preserving muscular volume.

➢ You can begin anytime – no major planning or preparation needed. It is best to consult with your medical doctor before beginning any dieting regimen, but other than that, there is no other planning needed. You can begin as early as tomorrow!

➢ Your body's insulin levels become nearly dormant and remain very low during fasting which causes your body to rely on using body fat for energy. When your insulin levels are low, your body is in peak fat-burning mode.

➢ Very easy way to lose weight! No more crazy fad diets with crazy limitations or requirements – even better, with intermittent fasting you are more likely to keep the weight off!

➢ You will have insane amounts of natural energy – sans the jitters and mid-day crashes!

➢ You will perform better physically and mentally with increased clarity, alertness, focus, and peak physical conditioning.

➢ Freedom from being a slave to counting calories, reading nutrition labels, taking weight loss/diet supplements, etc.

Cons:

Note: Most of the cons listed are issues that happen early on in the intermittent fasting routine. These things happen as a person's body adjusts to the fasting process. While many of the following issues happen during 3 or more days' worth of fasting, they have also been known to effect people on 1 and 2 day fasts as well. Symptoms will vary from person to person.

➢ An obsession with food during fasting periods can tend to lead to binging on food when you are able to feed again. Strong self-discipline is a must until your body and mind adjusts to the fasting/feeding cycles.

➢ When women begin intermittent fasting, even short durations of fasting can lead to hormonal changes which can induce adult acne, irregular menstrual cycles, mood swings, roller coaster-like changes to metabolic rate, and depression.

➢ Insomnia can affect both sexes, but particularly women. The insomnia occurs due to the stimulation of hypocretin neurons, which can provoke alertness and wakefulness, making it very difficult to sleep. The good news is that once your body gets used to fasting, your sleep cycles will even out and the insomnia will dissipate.

➢ Dependence on coffee, energy drinks, and other sources of caffeine due to lack of energy.

➢ During your first few fasts, as your body is becoming used to the changes in your eating habits, it will go through Pavlov Reflexes (also referred to as Conditional Reflex). This is when your body automatically responds during specific times of the day when it is used to being fed. For example, you may be used to eating at each day at 8:00 A.M., 12:00 P.M., and 5:00 P.M. During fasting, when these times roll around, your body may begin to signal you through hunger pangs, cravings, growling stomach, cramps, mood swings, and other symtoms as a way to remind you to eat. Conditional reflexes can encourage people to cheat during fasting, break their fasting cycle, or overeat as soon as they are able.

Intermittent Fasting vs. Alternate Day Fasting

Those who find that they cannot overcome some of the challenges associated with intermittent fasting will often times opt for alternate day fasting.

You now know that intermittent fasting consists of fasting/feeding cycles that last from 16 to 48 hours at a time, with normal feeding on non-fast days. During fasts, only water and natural green tea is allowed.

Alternate day fasting is similar to intermittent fasting in that it requires fasting/feeding cycles with fasting durations which last 16 to 48 hours at a time. The difference is that during the alternate day fast, instead of being only allowed water and natural green tea, you can continue to eat. You eat at a very restricted calorie rate, 300 to 500 calories for women; 400 to 600 calories for men.

Alternate day fasting is obviously the easier choice. However, the results may not be as remarkable or as quick as with intermittent fasting. Intermittent fasting burns fat at a much faster rate due to insulin levels remaining dormant during the fast.

It is recommended that you begin with intermittent fasting – see how you do, how well and how quickly you adjust. If after a month or two - I would definitely try to give it at least 8 weeks- you find that intermittent fasting is too difficult, or if you find that you can't help but cheat on fast days, or find yourself overeating on feed days, then alternate day fasting may be the answer for you.

On the other hand, there is more work involved in alternate day fasting. For instance, you are constantly counting calories, both on fast and feed days. With intermittent fasting, there is no need to count calories, although you can if you like. It is actually better if you do not count calories. On feed days (also referred to as feast days) you are pretty much able to eat as you wish, and you *want* to eat well so that the fasting/feeding cycles are very dramatic – you want your body flip-flopping from extreme to extreme. This will trick your body into thinking it is starving, which will lead to intense fat burning.

Both types of fasting/feeding regimens offer numerous long-term health benefits. Both options burn fat, promote weight loss, rid the body of toxins, and offer disease preventative and ailment-curing properties – however with intermittent fasting you receive all of the above benefits and more at a much faster rate.

Take a look at the following table for a side-by-side glance at the differences between intermittent fasting and alternate day fasting:

Intermittent Fasting vs. Alternate Day Fasting	
Intermittent Fasting	**Alternate Day Fasting**
* No planning or preparation required	* Easier for beginners
* Much faster results	* Better for those who tend to binge eat
* Can start immediately	* Better for those with lack of self-discipline
* 50% reduction in grocery/food bills	* No strict "NO FOOD" days
* Risk of binge eating	* 15% to 30% reduction in grocery/food bills
* Need self-discipline to not cheat on fast days	* Slower results
* Water/natural green tea fasting ONLY	* Restricted calorie fasting
* Intense fat-burning cycles	* Planning and preparation needed
* Long-term health benefits	* Long-term health benefits
* Strict "NO FOOD" fasting	* Able to eat 7 days per week.

Overall, I believe in the results and benefits of intermittent fasting. Although some people prefer alternate day fasting, I recommend starting out with an intermittent fasting plan, such as the wonderful 5:2 Diet. When you begin, do your very best to give it at least 8 weeks and if you find it to be just too difficult, you can always switch. However, you may decide to stick with it once you see how amazing the results are in as little as 8 weeks!

Part 2: Living the 5:2 Lifestyle

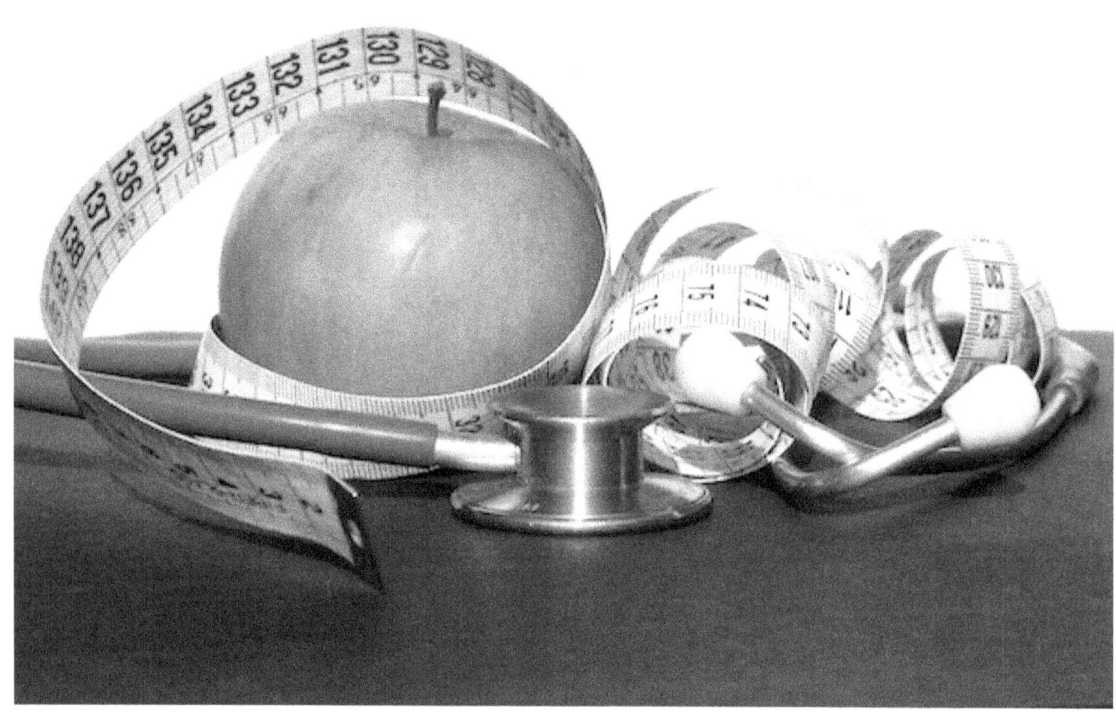

The 5:2 Diet: What it is, What it Does, and is it for YOU?

What it is

First off, I disagree with the term 'diet' when referring to the 5:2 Diet because you will find that 5:2 is much more a **lifestyle** then a "diet." The 5:2 Diet, sometimes written as the 5/2 Diet is a form of intermittent fasting. It involved intervals of fasting and feeding days. With the 5:2 Diet, you follow:

> ➢ **5 Feed-Days**
> ➢ **2 Fast-Days (non-consecutive days)**

Look at the following example of a typical 5:2 Diet Week:

Example of a Typical 5:2 Diet Week

SUNDAY	MONDAY	TUESDAY	WEDNESDAY	THURSDAY	FRIDAY	SATURDAY
Feed	Fast	Feed	Feed	Fast	Feed	Feed

It's as simple as that. The 5:2 Diet uses a medium duration of fasts on the intermittent fasting spectrum – 24 hours. Remember, with intermittent fasting the fasting duration ranges in length from 16 hours to 48 hours.

With the 5:2 Diet, you have two choices:

> ➢ **2-day severely Restricted-Calorie Fasts** (Conventional 5:2 Method)
> ➢ **2-day "NO Food" Fasts – Allows water and natural green tea ONLY**

The conventional 5:2 Diet follows the restricted calorie fasting; however, more and more people are choosing to opt for the no-food fasts, as they are finding that the results are much quicker. For the remaining 5 days, you are pretty much able to eat as you please, within reason. It is important that you eat well; you want for there to be a dramatic difference between your feeding and fasting days. With restricted calorie fasting, you are to reduce your calorie intake to 1/4 (25%) of your normal daily calorie consumption, which is on average, no more than 500 calories per day for women and 600 calories per day for men. Again, restricted calorie fasting is the conventional method for the 5:2 Diet, and it is better for those individuals who are not able to maintain successful no-food fasting. However, you still have the option of no-food fasts. If you try both types of fasts you will find that even though it may not seem like it on paper, there is a BIG difference between a 500-calorie restricted calorie fast and a no-food fast. With a no-good fast you are burning fat at a much faster rate. You lose more weight, and you lose it quicker. The short- and long-term health benefits are more noticeable and happen faster. 2-day no-food fasts are truly the way to go – as long as you don't find yourself binge-eating during your feed days.

Remember: You're not a bear preparing for hibernation! There is no reason to over-indulge in food. Believe me when I say that your first fast may seem impossible. It may seem like your body will never get use to the fasts. It may seem like you're pouring every ounce of your energy into willing yourself away from the refrigerator – however, it DOES get easier! After a couple of months, you won't believe how simple the fasts become for you! You will breeze through the 2-day no-food fasts and feel great.

8 weeks. Give yourself 8 weeks of the 5:2 Diet with no-food fasts. That is only eight fasting cycles! Then try to set a goal for another 8 weeks, for a total of 16 fasting cycles. If after that you still find yourself struggling to get through the fasts. or you find yourself overeating during feed days because you feel deprived during the fasting cycles, THEN you can begin to switch over to restricted calorie fasts.

Another option for those who find no-food fasts to be too hard is to alternate between no-food fasting and restricted calorie fasting during every other fasting cycle. For example:

Week One: 5-Day Feed with 2-Day NO-Food Fast
Week Two: 5-Day Feed with 2-Day Restricted Calorie Fast
Week Three: 5-Day Feed with 2-Day NO-Food Fast
Week Four: 5-Day Feed with 2-Day Restricted Calorie Fast
(All on non-consecutive days)

Rest assured, you WILL find a personalized 5:2 fasting/feeding cycle that works for you.

Working with Restricted Calorie Fasting

Even though you have the option of no-food fasting, for the rest of this book we will be focusing on the traditional method of the 5:2 Diet: restricted calorie fasting.

The 5:2 Diet is by far the easiest type of diet in which to participate. That being said, there still may be times you find yourself becoming frustrated with the diet. If you ever get discouraged, just put the whole 5:2 Diet into perspective. Compare it to some of the other diets you have tried in the past. The 5:2 Diet is so incredibly convenient and easy! Take a look at the following 5:2 Diet highlights:

- ✓ Super easy and convenient

- ✓ No preparation or planning necessary

- ✓ Count calories only 2 days per week

- ✓ The diet is only 2 days per week – the other five days you are free to eat normally

- ✓ Burn fat faster! Burn more calories!

- ✓ Major short- and long-term health benefits

- ✓ Dramatic results quickly

- ✓ The weight comes off quickly and is easy to keep off!

- ✓ NO pills, supplements, injections, nasty-tasting shakes, or other special requirements

These are only a few of the major highlights of the 5:2 diet! The one that I want you to focus on is the highlight that states: ***The diet is only 2 days per week – the other five days you are free to eat normally.*** Think about that statement for a moment. Have you ever been on a diet regimen where all the work goes into just two days per week? Think about your most recent diet attempt – how many days did the diet require from you? Did you have to take a certain type of food, a pill or injection, intense exercise, weigh-ins, count calories or points, cook complex recipes, and bend over backwards just to see a little benefit? Most diets require some type of effort from you seven days per week – some five days per week, but how many diets only require effort two days per week? ONLY ONE - The 5:2 Diet! Are you up for it? Once you experience 5:2 and see how convenient it is and that it actually works – you will *never* turn to another diet method again! Simply put, the 5:2 Diet works – and it WILL work for you!

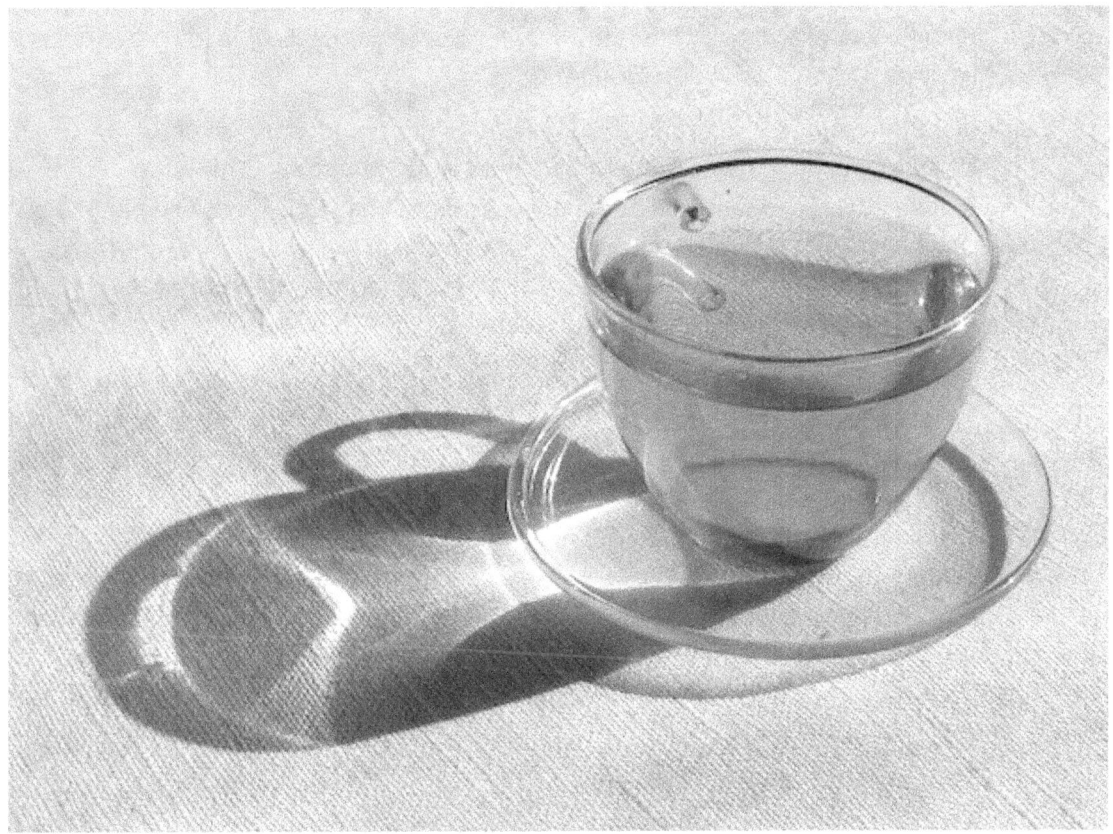

What it Does

Intermittent fasting, such as the 5:2 Diet, has been studied and scrutinized by doctors, scientists, nutritionists, and the like. Study after study has been completed on the weight loss and health results gained from short fasting cycles, and the one conclusion that keeps being determined through clinical studies and trials is that intermittent fasting works! A study was recently done with mice where they were tested on the benefits of the 5:2 Diet, in particularly, restricted calorie fasting. The results showed that the mice following the 5:2 Diet lived 47% longer than mice not on the diet. In New Mexico in 2012, a human 5:2 Diet study took place and after just 8 weeks on the 5:2 Diet, every participant stated that they felt better, looked better, they all lost weight, they had more energy, were able to focus better and many mentioned that the "foggy" tired feeling that had plagued their minds lifted. The study also showed that their overall health and vitality had remarkably improved.

There is something about fasting that almost makes it seem too good to be true – but it isn't!

Those who have tried crash diets or fad diets before know that these diets fail within the first 2 weeks to one month because the dieter usually burns out. Most crash and fad diets require skipping meals or cutting out certain food products altogether, and many of these diets are also too complicated or take up too much of the dieter's time. The 5:2 Diet works because it tricks the body out of storing fat. Through fasting/feeding cycles the body is thrust into "repair mode" and instead of producing new cells, it begins repairing old ones, which uses up a lot more energy. Now, instead of storing fat, the body begins burning it.

Restricted calorie fasting lowers the body's insulin levels significantly, and the body begins burning fat for its energy supply instead, using up the existing fat stores. This is why the 2-day fast (two non-consecutive days) is so perfect for weight loss. The 2-day fast is really what the 5:2 Diet is. When you fast, your insulin levels stay low – it's when your insulin levels are low that you begin burning fat like crazy. The more active you are during your fast, the more fat and calories you burn. That in turn leads to more weight loss.

Even if you hate exercising, if you want to see the fat melt off your body quickly, then hit the cardio during your fast days. It is absolutely worth it! Many people worry that they will be too tired and weak to exercise during fasting days. Not the case! You are not on a 3-week fast, its 2 days! Besides, people usually feel weak and tired during fasting if they are dehydrated. Remember: water is crucial to the success of the 5:2 Diet. You must stay hydrated during fasting! The more active you are, the more water you will need, but you should at least drink a gallon of water per day during fasting. If you keep yourself hydrated, you will actually find that you are able to work out more intensely. You will find that you have an abundance of raw, natural energy during fasting. If you can commit yourself to at least 45-minutes of cardio on each fasting day, then you will see results even faster!

The 5:2 Diet and You:

Now that you are ready to get started, there are a few things you need to know. It is time to personalize 5:2 to fit YOU! Read on for some important information you'll want to know as you begin the 5:2 lifestyle!

Getting Started

There is no planning or preparation needed to begin the 5:2 Diet. If you're like me, you plan for everything anyways, even when planning is not necessary. I feel that in order to truly give yourself the best head start possible, you should at least put a little thought into how you can make 5:2 work for you and fit into your lifestyle. Remember, the beauty of 5:2 is that it adapts to your schedule and molds itself to form around your life. Let's talk about how you can prepare to make sure you are setting yourself up for nothing less than optimum weight loss, health, and outstanding results.

Consult Your Doctor

Though we mentioned this before, it is important enough to mention again. Before you begin this or any other diet, it is a good idea to talk about the diet with your doctor to make sure that it is appropriate for you. Many doctors recommend intermittent fasting diets such as 5:2 because of the scientific backing. These types of diets are, for the most part, widely supported by scientists, nutritionists, and medical doctors alike. Therefore getting the A-OK from your doctor should be incredibly easy! If you have any health conditions that require you to eat a certain type of meals, or restricted diet, it is of vital importance that you speak with your doctor before beginning 5:2. Your doctor may have a simple alternative or a method that allows you to be able to safely partake in the diet.

In reality, many of us skip the trip to the doc. Perhaps it's because we don't want to be told that we *can't* try a diet or maybe we don't have health insurance or maybe we don't have time to make an appointment. However we try to justify not consulting our doctor, it really is a very critical step in beginning any new diet. Many people become so excited about the possibilities a new diet may hold that they decide to jump in first and ask questions later.

Now, this diet *is* very safe, fasting is one of the healthiest, most natural things you can do for your body. Every time you fast, you are cleansing your body and ridding it of toxins – and that is beneficial in so many ways. However, it is still better to be safe than sorry, and even if you do not have any conditions that could interfere with the diet, it is still worth the trip to the doctor. Besides, your doc may have some valuable insight to offer that will help you during this diet. Maybe they have a creative method to help get you through fasting. Maybe they have a great idea about how to spread out your limited calories during your 2-day fast. Who knows, your doctor may hold the key to what will help you be successful in this diet. Remember, intermittent fasting diets have been studied for years by nutritionists and scientists. It's likely that your doctor, being a part of health science, has also studied intermittent fasting diets along the way, so ask him or her for inspiration and guidance.

Setting Your Weight Loss Goals

This is a very important step. People usually are more successful in diets when they have goals to follow and milestones to hit. Setting goals is a way to challenge yourself. It is a way to hold yourself accountable. When you set a goal, it's as if you are telling yourself that failing is not an option. If you don't meet a goal, that usually gives you the will and motivation to crush the next goal. Some people are scared to set weight loss goals for themselves. They are afraid that if they do not meet their goal that they will just figure the diet's a flop or too hard, or they will decide that they just don't have what it takes, and they will give up.

I cannot speak for everyone, and sadly in some cases failing a goal or milestone does have such a negative impact on a person that they decide to quit. You have to give yourself the benefit of the doubt; you have to promise yourself from the start that QUITTING IS NOT AN OPTION – even if you don't meet one of your goals. I tell clients all the time that it's our failures in dieting that make us stronger. Failure builds character; it is through failure that a person decides who they want to be. It is a moment of fight or flight. When trying to lose weight, it is important that you remain strong, determined, and unwilling to give up. During a diet, you may not hit *every* goal, but you need to acknowledge that as a possibility from the beginning.

If you meet a goal, reward yourself with something small: a new outfit to go along with your ever-slimming body, a massage, a mani-pedi, or get a babysitter so you can have the night off. However you choose to reward yourself is entirely up to you - just make sure you do reward yourself in some way!

If you miss a goal, DON'T PANIC! Try to figure out what went wrong and learn from it. Thank yourself for the effort and make a promise to yourself to do your best to meet the next goal. When coming up with your goals, keep them small and reachable!

A few examples of reachable goals are:

"For the week of _____, my goal is to lose 2 lbs."
"My goal this week is to do 1 hour of cardio on Monday, Wednesday, and Friday."
"My goal this week is to walk a total of 5 miles by Saturday."

A few examples of unrealistic goals are:

"For the week of _____, my goal is to lose 10 lbs."
"My goal this week is to walk 8 miles per day, every day."
"My goal for my 2-day fast this week is to eat no more than 100 calories each day."

Now, can you understand why the second group of goals is unrealistic? Note: I say "unrealistic" not "impossible," except for the first one – it is impossible to lose 10 pounds per week in a healthy manner. These three goals are unrealistic because they are too hard.

Again, you cannot safely lose 10 pounds per week. With a restricted calorie fast you can expect to lose anywhere between 1 – 3 lbs. per week. Of course, every person is different. Men seem to lose weight at a faster rate than women; some women lose weight faster than other women. You could have two women or two men very similar in make-up (height, weight, activity levels, etc.) and they will each lose weight at different rates.

Weight loss tends to be slower in the beginning as your body, metabolic rate, insulin and blood sugar levels adjust to the diet. Do not fret if for the first 2 or 3 weeks you are only losing a pound, if even, per week. It is worth the wait, believe me! Soon, the weight will begin melting off and you may find yourself losing 3 to 4 lbs. per week! Therefore, when setting your first month of goals, keep this in mind.

The next goal of walking 8 miles per day, every day, is also unrealistic. This is partially because Americans are busy, busy people. I don't know anyone who has enough time on their hands to walk 8 miles per day! Most of us have jobs, kids, and so many other priorities that we are lucky to get in a 30-minute workout each day - and that's being generous! When setting exercise goals, think about how much extra time you have and set workout goals that will fit into that time. Also, set achievable workouts. If you haven't exercised in years, it's probably best not to set a workout goal of *60 minutes on the treadmill at a 15% incline and a speed of 5.5mph*. Baby steps. Instead, set a goal such as *20 minutes on the treadmill at a 3% incline and a speed of 2.0mph*. This is a much easier goal to achieve. You can then gradually set tougher workout goals for yourself the more you exercise.

The third goal is the most important one to cover. You are allowed during feed days a MAXIMUM of 2,000 calories for women, 2,400 calories for men. However, not everyone should be consuming the MAXIMUM amount of calories each day. We use 2,000/2,400 calories in 5:2 as a CEILING ONLY. Depending on body type, age, and other factors your suggested daily caloric intake will most certainly differ. Let's begin discussing how you can go about calculating the accurate amount of calories you should be consuming each day.

Determining Daily Caloric Intake

The amount of daily calories that you should be consuming really depends on four different factors:

- **Gender**
- **Height**
- **Weight**
- **Age**
- **Daily Activity Level**

Gender: Men are supposed to consume more calories than women. This is based on several factors, including that men tend to be taller than women and possess more muscle mass.

Height, Weight, and Age: These three factors are also very important in determining how many calories you should consume daily due to the following:

- ✓ The taller you are, the more calories you need.

- ✓ As you age, you begin burning fat and calories at a slower rate as your metabolism begins to slow down, therefore the amount of calories you should consume on a daily basis decreases.

- ✓ The more you weigh, the higher your daily caloric requirement is.

Activity Level: I am sure you can easily understand why activity level influences daily caloric intake, but humor me as I explain anyways!

The more active you are, the higher daily caloric intake you require. For instance, if you have a desk job and don't exercise at all, your calorie needs will be much less than the person with a physically demanding position at work who works out four days per week.

Now, taking in the above factors you will need to determine two things to determine your Daily Caloric Needs:

- ✓ **Your BMR:** This stands for your Basal Metabolic Rate. BMR determines the minimum daily caloric intake needed for a RESTING person.

- ✓ **Your TDEE:** This stands for your Total Daily Energy Expenditure; it evaluates how active you are each day, providing a rough estimate of a daily caloric intake that will meet your individual needs.

Let's take a closer look at each.

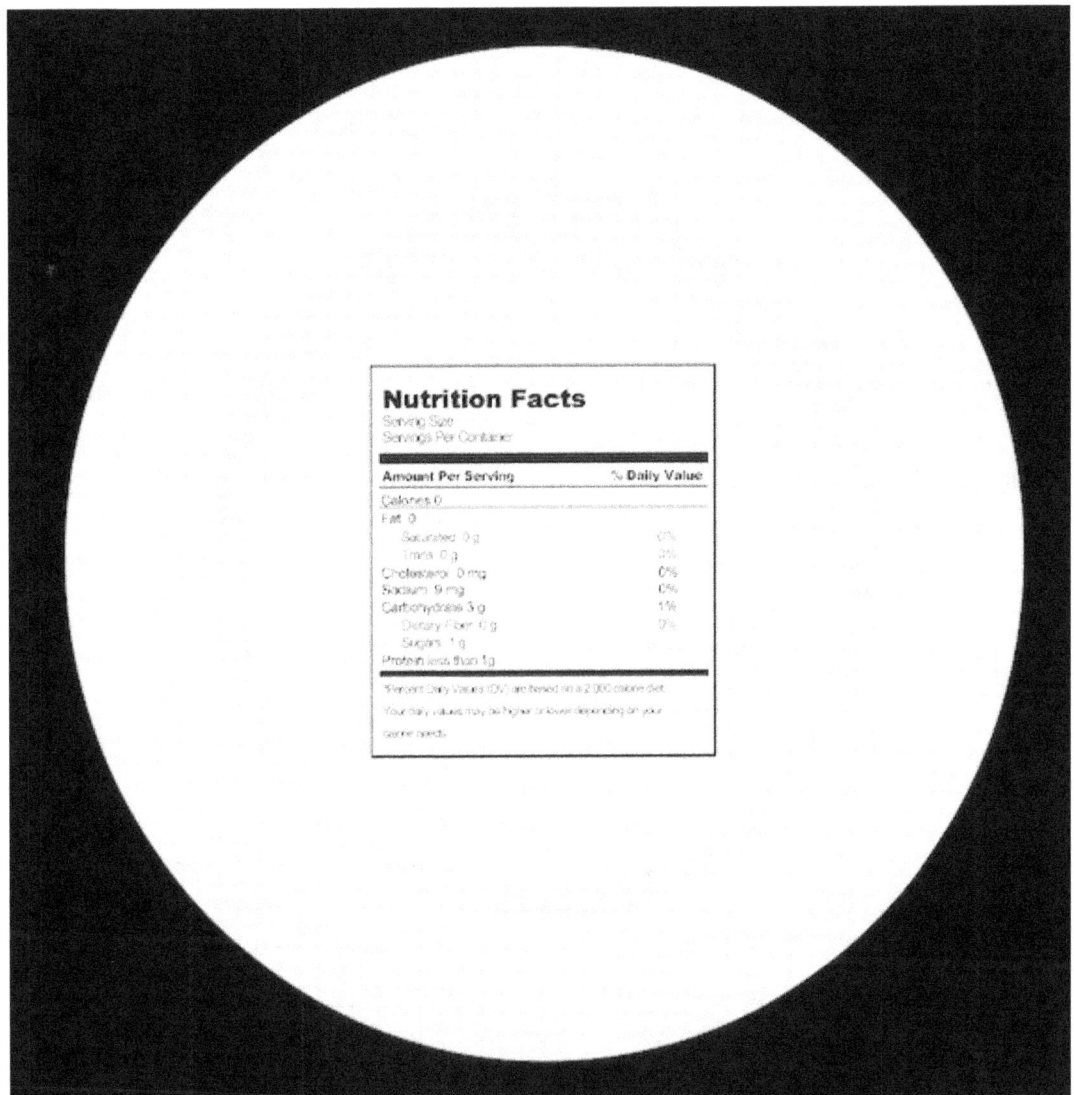

BMR (Basal Metabolic Rate)

Your body uses energy all day, every day no matter what you are doing – it doesn't matter if you are sitting on the couch watching TV or running a marathon, your body uses energy either way. BMR is responsible for nearly 70% of the calories you're your body expends each and every day. To put it simply, your BMR tells you how many calories your body would burn if you were to stay in bed all day long. Your BMR will help you determine your metabolic rate as well as the number of calories you need to burn daily in order for you to lose, gain or maintain your weight.

Have you ever noticed how most teenagers can eat all day long, sleep all day, and not do much of anything, yet stay super thin? This is because their BMR is so high. As you age, your BMR decreases. You can no longer eat what you want without it dropping to your hips and sticking to them. On the upside, there is a secret to keeping your BMR rate high the older you get. The answer to your prayers involves regularly scheduled cardio workouts! Cardiovascular conditioning will keep your BMR high and your calories burning quickly! A persons BMR is based on several different factors, such as:

- **Genetics:** Some people are born with faster metabolisms than others.

- **Gender:** Men tend to have faster metabolisms and burn more fat and calories than women.

- **Weight and Age:** Younger people tend to have faster metabolisms that older people. Scientifically speaking, your BMR drops 2% each decade after 20 years of age. The more you weigh, the faster your BMR. In fact, people who are obese typically have 25 to 30% faster metabolisms than people who are underweight or at their ideal weight.

- **Body Surface Area and Body Fat Percentage:** Your body surface area is determined by your weight and height. Someone who is 6 feet 3 inches and weighs 340lbs. is going to have a larger body surface are than a person who is 5 foot 4 inches and weight 110lbs. A person with a larger body surface area will have a faster metabolism than someone with a smaller body area.

- **Health:** A body that is physically healthy will have a better BMR than a body suffering from poor health, malnutrition, disease, etc.

- **Internal/External Body Temperatures:** The higher your internal body temperature, the faster your metabolism and the higher your BMR. Believe it or not, your external body temperature also plays a role in your BMR rate. When you feel cold, your BMR increases in order for your body to warm itself up and maintain its internal temperature. Heat exposure does not have much of an impact on your BMR, unless you are exposed to heat for an extended period of time – in this case, your BMR will increase.

- **Activity Levels:** The more you exercise, the more your BMI increases in order to accommodate the lean tissue you are developing through physical activity. Lean tissue is more taxing on your metabolism that fat tissue – so the more you exercise, the more lean tissue is built, the more your BMR increases, the more calories you burn (even while sleeping)!

TDEE (Total Daily Energy Expenditure)- Caloric Maintenance Level

Your TDEE is the total number of calories your body expends in a 24-hour period, which includes all activity. TDEE is also considered to be your caloric "maintenance" level. It provides you with the number of calories you need to take in each day in order to maintain your current weight. The basic definition of your caloric maintenance level is:

When Calories IN = Calories OUT, You have reached your Caloric Maintenance Level

For example, if you burn 2200 calories per day (this includes all activity – walking into work, vacuuming your house, playing with your kids, working out, etc.), then you need to have a daily calorie intake of 2200 calories. This way the amount of calories going in and coming out are equal, they cancel each other out, so your weight will remain the same.

If more calories are going out then coming in, you will lose weight.

If more calories are coming in then going out, then you will gain weight.

Caloric maintenance levels vary from person to person, but on average, maintenance levels range from 2,000-2,100 calories per day for women and 2,700-2,900 calories per day for men. The more active you are the more calories you need. Let's take athletes for example; it is not unheard of for athletes to have a daily maintenance level of over 3,000 calories. In fact, it is quite normal. For instance, U.S. Gold Olympic Swimmer, Michael Phelps, stated in a previous interview that he maintains a daily caloric intake of 12,000 calories! He admitted that his recommended daily caloric intake was between 8,000 to 10,000 calories, but that he has found that he needs even more in order to maintain his weight and to endure his levels of activity.

Once you determine your TDEE, or maintenance level, you will be able to figure out how many calories need to be decreased or increased from your maintenance level in order for you to be able to lose or gain weight. Your maintenance level is by far the most important factor when trying to lose/maintain/gain weight. If you know your maintenance level, you will have a better chance of meeting your desired weight goals.

Calculating your BMR and TDEE (Caloric Maintenance Level)

There are a few methods that can be used in determining your caloric maintenance level. Whichever method you choose, each will give you an accurate result tailored around your own individual needs.

The first method is most popular by many people because it is the easiest method to use, take a look:

The Body Weight Method

(Based on Total Body Weight)

This method is not as precise as the others because it does not take into account some factors such as age, gender, or physical activity, and it gives you a high/low range as oppose to a set number, so you have to keep your daily caloric intake within that range. However, even though the results may not be as specific as the other methods, the range it gives is accurate. Many people prefer the range this method provides because it gives them more leeway within the 5:2 Diet. To find your caloric maintenance level, the numbers in the table are to be used as your multipliers. The results offer a low to high range.

For Fat Loss:	12-13 calories per lb. of body weight.
For Maintenance:	15-16 calories per lb. of body weight.

For Weight Gain:	17-19 calories per lb. of body weight.

Take your current weight and multiply by both numbers.

If your goal is to LOSE weight:

Current Weight x 12 = Low range of calories needed to lose weight
Current Weight x 13 = High range of calories needed to lose weight

If your goal is to MAINTAIN weight:

Current Weight x 15 = Low range of calories needed to maintain current weight
Current Weight x 16 = High range of calories needed to maintain current weight

If your goal is to GAIN weight:

Current Weight x 17 = Low range of calories needed to gain weight
Current Weight x 19 = High range of calories needed to gain weight

Let's try one:

If you want to LOSE weight and you currently weigh 125 lbs.:

125 lbs. x 12 = 1500 (this is your LOW end range maintenance level)
125lbs x 13 = 1625 (this is your HIGH end range maintenance level)

Caloric Maintenance Level = 1500 – 1625
Our example person must remain somewhere within these numbers to lose weight.

When trying to figure out where you should fall between these two numbers, it is up to you to consider all necessary factors such as age, gender, and activity level. For instance:

- Females tend to have a slower metabolism than males, so this means that women should keep to the lower end; men toward the higher end of their maintenance level range.

- The older you are the slower your metabolism, so stick to the lower end of the range. Remember, after the age of 20, your BMR decreases a little more each decade that passes. If you really want to do the math, it's 2% decrease per decade.

Let's now move on to the second method.

The Harris-Benedict Equation

(BMR Based on Total Body Weight)

This method is a bit more complicated, but has a much higher level of accuracy because it makes you take into account all of the factors that lead to your recommended caloric maintenance level. The Harris-Benedict Method is a caloric formula which implements factors such as gender, age, height, weight, and activity level as a basis for determining your BMR (Basal Metabolic Rate).

This method is much more precise than the first method, because it factors in more than just body weight.

HOWEVER, this method DOES NOT take in to account lean body mass, therefore this method may not provide as much accuracy for those who are exceptionally muscular or extremely obese.

In those who are very muscular, this method will underestimate daily calorie needs and for those who are very obese, this method with overestimate daily calorie needs.

To find your caloric maintenance level using the Harris-Benedict Equation method, refer to the method on the next page.

Meet Paul. Paul is going to help us throughout the Harris-Benedict Equation Method.

Let's first begin by getting to know Paul:

Paul is a **male.**
Paul is **38 years-old.**
Paul's current weight is **224lbs.**
Paul's height is **73-inches.**
Paul's activity level is **Moderate Activity**

In order to figure out Paul's recommended caloric maintenance level, we first need to calculate his BMR:

Note: **BMR = Basal Metabolic Rate; w = weight; h = height**
This method uses the metric system:
1-inch = 2.54cm
2.2 pounds = 1kg

The Harris-Benedict Equation (BMR Based on Total Body Weight)	
Formulas used to determine BMR:	
Men:	BMR = 66 + (13.7 x **w** in kg.) + (5 x **h** in cm.) – (6.8 x current age)
Women:	BMR = 655 + (9.6 x **w** In kg.) + (9.6 x **h** in cm.) – (4.7 x current age)

First, convert Paul's height and weight from imperial to metric.

Paul weighs **224lbs.** (224 / 2.2 = **101.8 kg**)

Paul's height is **73-inches.** (73 x 2.54 = **185.4 cm**)

Now, using the following formula, find Paul's BMR:
BMR = 66 + (1394.7 + 927) – (258.4)
66 + (2321.7 – 258.4) = 2129.3 (rounded to 2129)
Paul's BMR = 2129

Now that we know Paul's BMR, we can now calculate his TDEE, by multiplying his BMR by the Activity Level Multiplier that bests describes him, in the chart below.

Calculating TDEE	
Activity Level	**Multiplier**
Sedentary *(little to no exercise; desk job)*	Sedentary = BMR x 1.2
Light Activity *(Light exercise/activity 1-3 days/wk)*	Light Activity = BMR x 1.375
Moderate Activity *(Mod. exercise/activity 3-5 days/wk)*	Moderate Activity = BMR x 1.55
Heavy Activity *(Intense exercise/activity 6 days/wk)*	Heavy Activity = BMR x 1.725
Excessive Activity *(Intense daily exercise/ physically demanding job or exercise multiple times/day)*	Excessive Activity = BMR x 1.9

Let's find Paul's TDEE, by using the following formula:
Paul's BMR : **2129**
Paul's Activity Level is: **Moderate Activity**
The Activity Level Multiplier for Moderate Activity is: **1.55**

TDEE = BMR x Activity Level Multiplier
2129 x 1.55 = 3299.9 (rounded to 3300)
Paul's TDEE = 3301 (Caloric Maintenance Level)

Moving on to the final method...

The Katch-McArdle Formula

(BMR Based on Lean Body Mass/Weight)

This is the most accurate method of all for calculating your recommended caloric intake. It is only for those of you who have your body composition analyzed regularly and know the amount of lean body mass that your body contains.

In the Harris-Benedict Equation the formulas are different for men and women, because lean body mass is not a factor considered. Men tend to have more lean body mass than women, so the Harris-Benedict Equation makes up for that difference in the gender formulas. This method has the same formula for both men and women because lean body mass *is* part of the equation.

Meet Beth. Beth is going to help us throughout the Katch-McArdle Formula Method.

Let's first begin by getting to know Beth:
Beth is a **female**.
Beth is **24 years-old.**
Beth's Body Fat Percentage is **20%** (24lbs. Fat/ 96lbs. Lean)
Beth's Lean Body Mass is **96 lbs.**
Beth's height is **62-inches.**
Beth's activity level is **Light Activity**

First, convert Beth's Lean Body Mass from imperial to metric.
Beth's Lean Body Mass is **96 lbs. (43.6 kg.)**

Formula used to find Beth's BMR:

BMR (men and women) = 370 + (21.6 x lean body mass in kg.)

370 + (21.6 x 43.6) = Beth's BMR
370 + 941.76 = 1311.76 (rounded to 1312)
Beth's BMR = **1312 Calories/Day**

Finally, let's find Beth's TDEE.

To do so, multiply Beth's BMR by her Activity Level multiplier.

Formula used to find Beth's TDEE:

Beth's TDEE = Activity Level Multiplier x BMR

Beth's BMR is **1312**
Beth's Activity Level is **Light Activity**
Beth's Activity Level Multiplier is **1.375**

1.375 x 1312 = Beth's TDEE
1.375 x 1312 = 1804
Beth's TDEE = 1804 (Caloric Maintenance Level)

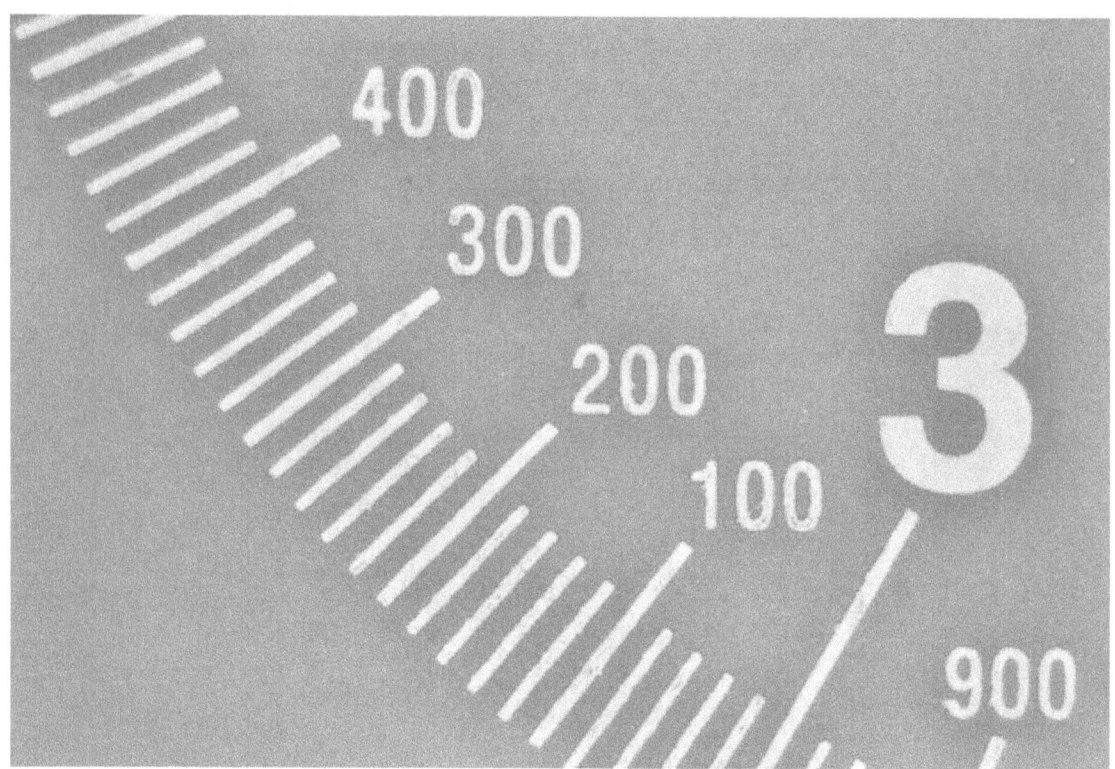

Caloric Deficit Threshold

Now, we are venturing into the area which most dieters wonder about.

How many calories should I eat if I am trying to lose weight?

We began answering this above by calculating your BMR and TDEE, however, there is another important area we should discuss and that is your Calorie Deficit (or the lowest amount of calories your body should intake on a daily basis to lose weight. When you discover your suggested maintenance level, you begin to use that number as a base for the amount of daily calories you consume. Relying on this maintenance level, you can lose weight in one of two ways:

- The first way is to eat a number of daily calories that are less than your maintenance level. The best way to do this is to learn your calorie deficit threshold.

- The second way you can lose weight is to eat at your daily maintenance level, but increase your activity level. This will make it so there are more calories coming out than going in, resulting in weight loss.

Calculating Your Calorie Deficit Threshold

The most common and simplest way to determine your calorie deficit threshold for weight loss is to cut your maintenance level calories by at least 500 calories but no more than 1,000 calories. If you cut your calories down too much, it could easily cause devastating health issues.

You want to lose weight, but you want to do it safely. What would be the point of losing a lot of weight and looking amazing, if you couldn't be around to enjoy it? ***KEEP IT SMART AND PLAY IT SAFE***.

If you cut your maintenance level down 500-1,000 calories, then you are destined for weight loss – there is no need to cut down by more than 1,000 calories.

Example:

Kim's TDEE (Maintenance Level) is: **1971 Calories/Day**

Kim's calorie deficit to lose weight is: **500**

1971 – 500 = 1471

Kim's calorie deficit threshold is: **1471 Calories/Day**

The second method that can be used to determine your calorie deficit threshold is to reduce your calories to 15 to 20% lower than your TDEE. This method is a little more individualized because it accounts for your body weight and TDEE as well.

Example:

Kim's TDEE is **1652**

Kim's calorie deficit to lose weight is **20% of TDEE = 330**

1652 – 330 = 1322

Kim's optimal caloric intake for weight loss is: **1322 Calories/Day**

During your fast days, you are to only consume a 1/4 (25%) of your feed day calorie intake.

As stated before, the average maintenance level for women is 2000-2100 calories per day; and for men, the average maintenance level is 2700-2900. For the sake of the 5:2 Diet:

- Women are recommended to follow a diet of no more than 2000 calories/day on their feed days and 500 calories/day on each fast day.

- Men are recommended to follow a diet of no more than 2400 calories/day on their feed day and 600 calories/day on each fast day.

If you prefer to figure out your ideal recommended calories per day by calculating your BMR and TDEE, then on feed days, you are to eat the number of calories suggested by your TDEE (your maintenance level) and on fast days, only eat 1/4 of those calories. The calorie deficit (decreasing your maintenance level calories by 20%) should ONLY be used on feed days as a way to gain an extra weight loss advantage. On fast days, you must only use 1/4 of the total calories you consume on feed days.

During the beginning, you'll want to stick to the maximum allowed calorie intake for your fasting cycle. If after a while, you decide to reduce the fasting calorie intake a bit, that's fine, but this should only be done after you have had at least 12 successful 2-day fasts. After you are a seasoned faster, you can begin to drop your calories a bit.

Maybe take it down, 50 to 100 calories at a time – but 100 calorie total for each day is not easy and it is not a realistic goal for someone just starting out on 5:2. When your body becomes used to fasting, then you can take it down to 100 or 200 calories, but only then! Once you are a 5:2 fasting pro, I highly recommend doing a no food 2-day fast (Remember: two non-consecutive days)at least once per month during one of your fasting cycles, you will burn more fat and calories and your body will go through a great detox – not to mention all of the amazing health benefits.

To wrap up: Set small, achievable goals – you will have a better chance of meeting your goals and less of a chance of setting yourself up for failure. This is also part of the brilliance of the 5:2 Diet – it is so easy that it's almost fail proof! You will meet more goals because of the convenience and simplicity of the diet! In the next step, we will discuss your *5:2 Diet Journal* – I will show you an easy way to set up weekly/monthly goals in your journal. Read on!

Is it for YOU?

Something about the 5:2 Diet caught your attention. Maybe you read a book on the subject, maybe your doctor mentioned it, maybe you researched the diet online, maybe you have heard others speaking of the diet at work or your local coffee shop.
No matter how you got here..you're here now, and it's time to decide if the 5:2 Diet is appropriate for you! There are several things you have to consider when trying to decide if 5:2 is right for you.

First, this diet really is safe and effective for almost anyone. However, proceed with caution and consult your doctor if any of the following situations apply to you as dramatic diet/nutritional changes could put you at risk for further health issues:

Pregnant or Breastfeeding: If you are currently pregnant or breastfeeding or are trying to become pregnant, a restricted-calorie diet can put your unborn or breastfeeding child at risk. It could also decrease your chances of conceiving.

Diabetic or Hypoglycemic: This one falls into the next category as well, but needs to be highlighted separately. If you are diabetic or hypoglycemic, a restricted-calorie diet could put you at risk for complications. Also during fasts, your insulin levels are very low which could also lead to putting your health at risk. It is highly recommended, for health reasons, that you do not partake in the 5:2 Diet or any fasting diet.

Medical/Restricted Diets due to Chronic Conditions: If you have a certain condition or illness that requires you to eat a certain diet, and doesn't allow for fasting, then 5:2 may not be the right choice. Remember – the bulk of this diet is centered around the 2-day fast (Remember: two non-consecutive days) – without that, it won't work. If you are on a medical or restricted diet, talk things over with your doctor. If he or she thinks that the 2-day fast won't put you at risk, then it may be worth trying – but NO diet is worth risking your well-being.

Lack of Self-Discipline: Fasting is not for everyone. While restricted calorie fasting is easier than no food fasting, it still takes commitment, hard work, and determination. You need to consider whether or not you have the willpower and self-discipline to make it through your fasting days. It is not worth going through the fast just to gorge on food as soon as you are able. Ask yourself the following questions:

Will I be able to make it two days on 500 calories or less?

Will I be able to make it two days without giving in to my cravings?

Will I be able to make it through the fast, and not begin overeating as soon as the next feed day rolls around?

Will I be able to remain strong and determined throughout the 2-day fast?

Will I become too moody, stressed out, or anxious if I interrupt my normal eating patterns?

Am I open to change?

Am I willing to adjust to new eating patterns?

Am I willing to endure hard work in order to look better, feel better, and live a longer and healthier life?

These are crucial questions to think about. Many people cannot sit through a 1-hour TV show without eating. Some people cannot make it through a hard day at work or a fight with their spouse without turning to food for comfort. Some people may be able to make it through the 2-day fast, only to binge eat as soon as they are able to feed.

You do not want to set yourself up for failure – you do not want to sabotage yourself. Only you truly know how much you are able to control yourself and how much you eat. If you think that fasting will only lead to binge eating, then another type of diet may be better for you.

That being said, I still encourage you to at least give it a whirl. Who knows? Maybe right now you are thinking, "No way, no how! I will never make it!" Than you make it through your first fast with ease and brilliance – you just might surprise yourself. So no – while you don't want to set yourself up for failure, you still owe it to yourself to see if you can do 5:2. If not, at least you tried!

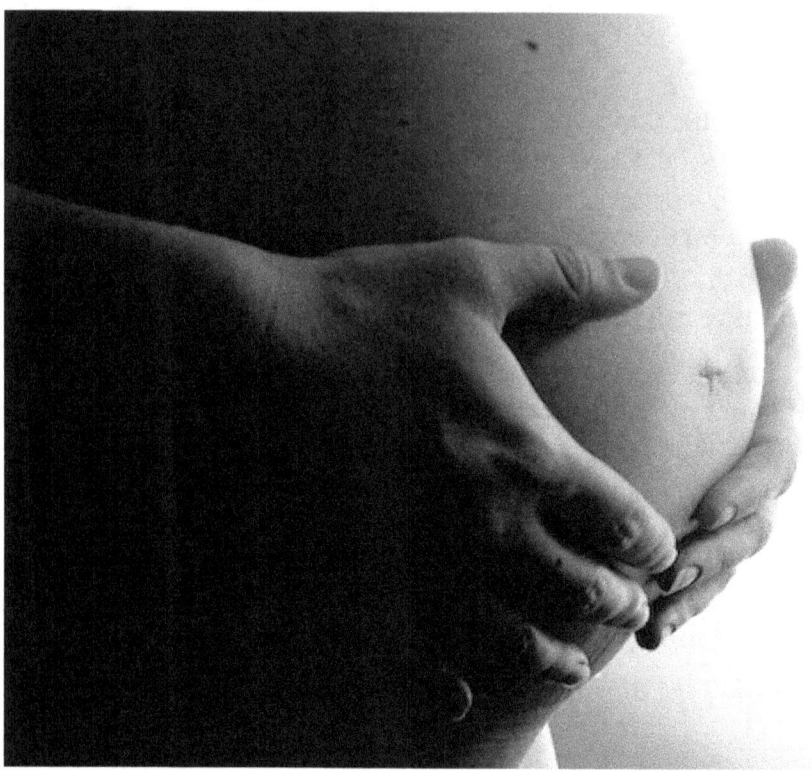

Creating Your 5:2 Diet Journal

The 5:2 Diet journal is soon to be your new best friend. The 5:2 Diet journal will become a very intimate part of your weight loss journey. It will see you through the trials and tribulations, celebrations and successes of your 5:2 experience. This journal will become hands-on inspiration for you and it will help you succeed during your weight loss journey!

I always recommend a diet journal. Use your journal every day, especially during your 2-days of fasting. Write anything you want – your hopes, wishes, dreams. Write about how you are feeling, what you think about the diet each week, write about what steps you can take to meet your goals. Write about ups and downs and everything in between. For many people, being on a diet is a very personal thing. They do not want to discuss it with anyone. This is where a journal becomes so important. You can talk everything out within your journal and never worry about being criticized or judged. A diet journal is the best way to release all of your emotions about the diet, and believe me – you will have plenty.

You will want to evaluate your journal often, and I encourage daily writing. You will also need to keep track of your progress both on a weekly and monthly basis. If, one day, you do not feel like writing much, I challenge you to at least write one sentence in your journal. The only thing is that your sentence must be positive. Maybe you can write out your favorite inspirational quote or a quick joke to make you laugh or something awesome that happened to you during the day. Even if you don't feel like writing out your thoughts and feelings about your weight loss, at least this sentence will keep you engaged and interacting with your journal. You do not want to skip a day of writing altogether, as that can easily lead to two days which can lead to one week, then a month, until your journal is at the bottom of a junk drawer. This journal WILL help you be successful during your 5:2 journey, so don't neglect it!

Take a look at the best way to create and set up your journal. Note: You can set up your journal any way you like; this is just a suggested way to format it. You want to make your journal as personalized and comfortable for you as possible. I encourage you to make the journal as much of an honest "YOU" as possible – many people keep their journals around for years to look back on for needed inspiration, so make sure when you look back on your journals five or ten years from now that you are looking back at a "portrait" of yourself!

Creating Your 5:2 Diet Journal

What you'll need:

- ✓ **5-Subject Notebook Journal with Inner Pockets** (it is best to opt for a college-ruled 3-ring paper binder. You can get a fancy binder or diary if you wish, but you will be going through quite a few journals, so you can save money with a standard journal).

- ✓ **Pens and Pencils; Markers and a Highlighter**

- ✓ **Personal Touches** (i.e., stickers, pictures, items of inspiration.

- ✓ **Scotch Tape and Glue** (glue sticks and hot glue guns work best)

- ✓ **Cloth measuring tape** (for body measurements)

- ✓ **Camera – optional** (for Before/After pictures)

- ✓ **Patience and a WHOLE LOTTA Honesty!**

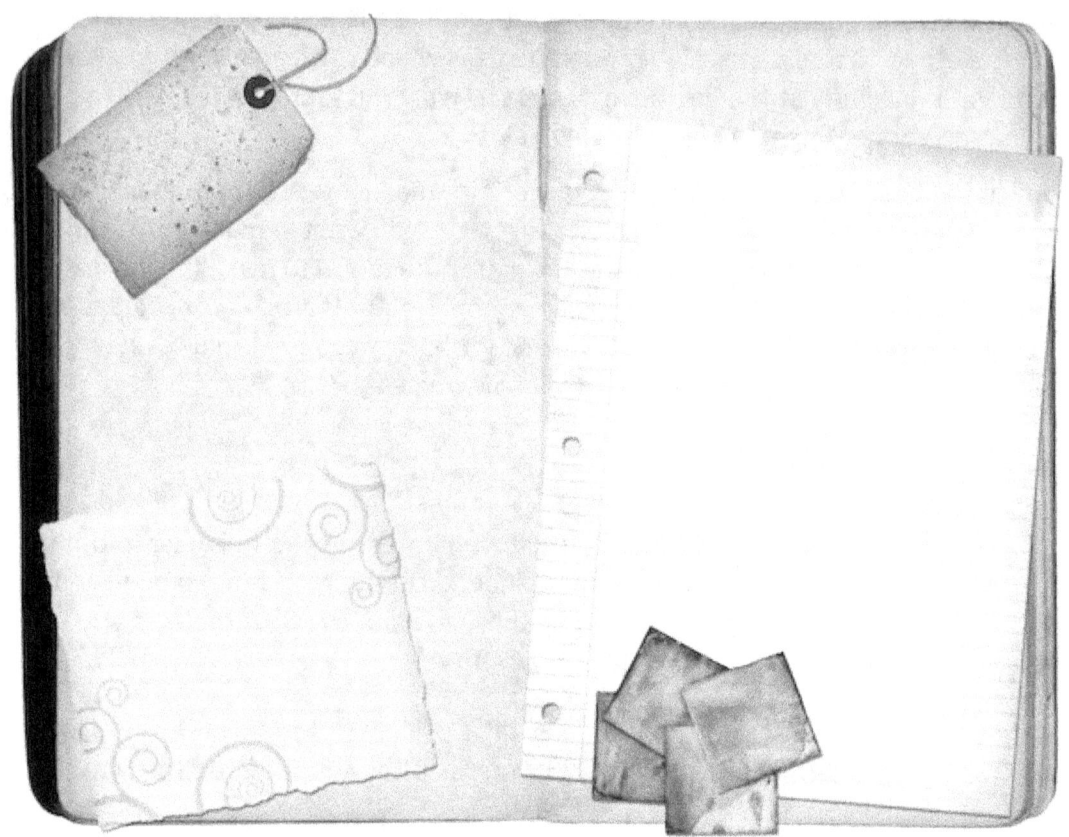

Instructions:

To begin, create a Fast/Feed Cycle Schedule: You can print out or buy a 12-month calendar (one that fits in the front inner pocket of your journal) and mark your feed/fast days so that you will always know where you are at during your feeding/fasting cycle and you will be able to plan ahead for future events. For example, say Christmas Day this year falls on a Thursday and Thursdays are typically one of your fast days – you do NOT want to find yourself fasting on Christmas with all the yummy food around. With the calendar you will be able dodge these kind of disasters!

Next, take your 5-subject journal and label each of the 5 sections with the following labels (Note: You can arrange the labels in whichever order you like or you can change the labels to any section titles you wish)**:**

1. **Goals:** Here is where you will write out your goals. It is best to cut your goal section into two parts. The first part should be "Weight Loss Goals". No matter what, you want to at least set a monthly weight loss goal. On a predetermined day once per month you will weigh yourself to see whether or not you reached your goal. The second part should be titled "Miscellaneous Goals". These can be exercise goals, calorie goals, body measurement or BMI goals, or whatever you wish. For these goals, you can set daily, weekly, monthly, or even yearly goals. The only rule is to keep them achievable; sure you want to challenge yourself – but only so

much. In this section you will also write down how you will reward yourself for meeting each goal (i.e., a nice dinner out, a new scarf, a new laptop case, etc.). Here is one good way to set up your goal section.

Monthly Weight Loss Goal			
Month: January		**Goal:** 10 lbs.	
Notes: A little tougher this month, but I am learning how to better divide up my fasting calories!			
Goal Achieved?	☑ Yes	☐	No
Reward: Cute shoes I saw at the department store!!!			
If goal was not achieved: How can I better meet my future goals?			

Monthly Weight Loss Goal			
Month: February		**Goal:** 12 lbs.	
Notes: Had a very hard time this month. Indulged a bit too much on Valentine's Day..			
Goal Achieved?	☐ Yes	☑	No
Reward: A new phone case (which I rewarded myself with anyways!)			
If goal was not achieved: How can I better meet my future goals?			
I will learn better ways to not overeat during the holidays. I need to teach myself how to better eat in moderation. I will do better next month!			

2. **Feeding/Fasting Daily Calorie Intake:** You will want to keep track of how many calories you eat, especially during your fasting cycle. You do not need to be detailed about your calorie intake during your feeding days, you just want to make sure you do not exceed 2000 calories/day for women or 2400 calories/day for men. You need to keep track only of your TOTAL daily feeding calories in order to ensure you are eating the correct amount of allowable calories. During fasting you are only allowed to eat **1/4** (25%) of your daily feeding calories. If you are a woman who eats 2,000 calories per day on her feeding days, then you are allowed a maximum of 500 calories per day on your fasting days. If you decrease your daily feeding calories to 1,600 calories per day then you will also have to decrease your allowed fasting calories to 400 calories per day. You will need to be very precise in counting your fasting calories.

Here is an example of how you can set up this section:

Daily Calorie Intake								
Month: January 2013								
	Week							
	Day	Sun.	Mon.	Tues.	Wed.	Thurs.	Fri.	Sat.
1	**Fast/Feed**	Feed	Fast	Feed	Feed	Fast	Feed	Feed
	Calorie Int.	2,000	500	2,000	2,000	500	2,000	2,000
	Day	Sun.	Mon.	Tues.	Wed.	Thurs.	Fri.	Sat.
2	**Fast/Feed**	Feed	Fast	Feed	Fast	Feed	Feed	Feed
	Calorie Int.	2,000	500	2,000	500	2,000	2,000	2,000
	Day	Sun.	Mon.	Tues.	Wed.	Thurs.	Fri.	Sat.
3	**Fast/Feed**	Feed	Feed	Fast	Feed	Fast	Feed	Feed
	Calorie Int.	2,000	2,000	500	2,000	500	2,000	2,000
	Day	Sun.	Mon.	Tues.	Wed.	Thurs.	Fri.	Sat.
4	**Fast/Feed**	Feed	Fast	Feed	Fast	Feed	Feed	Feed
	Calorie Int.	2,000	500	2,000	500	2,000	2,000	2,000
	Day	Sun.	Mon.	Tues.	Wed.	Thurs.		
5	**Fast/Feed**	Feed	Feed	Fast	Feed	Fast		
	Calorie Int.	2,000	2,000	500	2,000	500		

3. **Exercise Journal:** It is important, not only for weight loss but also for your health, that you get enough exercise. For this section, you will keep track of the type of exercise you did and the amount of time you exercised. You can take it even further and keep track of your calories lost. This is a good tool for holding yourself accountable in making sure you are getting enough exercise. Exercise doesn't have to be intense workouts, you can take a 20-minute walk or do 10 sit-ups. The goal here is that you are at least tracking some type of activity. Remember though - always try to do cardio workouts on your fasting days as you will burn more fat and calories. See the following example for a suggestion on how to set up your Exercise Journal section:

Exercise Journal		
Month/Year:	January 2013	
Date:	**Time Spent**	**Type of Exercise**
01/01/2013	15 minutes	Brisk Walk
01/02/2013	35 minutes	Treadmill (incline:4%/speed:2.5mph)
01/03/2013	20 minutes	P90X – abs and arms
01/05/2013	10 minutes	Resistance Bands
01/06/2013	60 minutes	Hiking
01/09/2013	25 minutes	Kickboxing Class
01/10/2013	30 minutes	Spin Class
01/12/2013	25 minutes	Free Weights/Abs
01/13/2013	60 minutes	Yoga

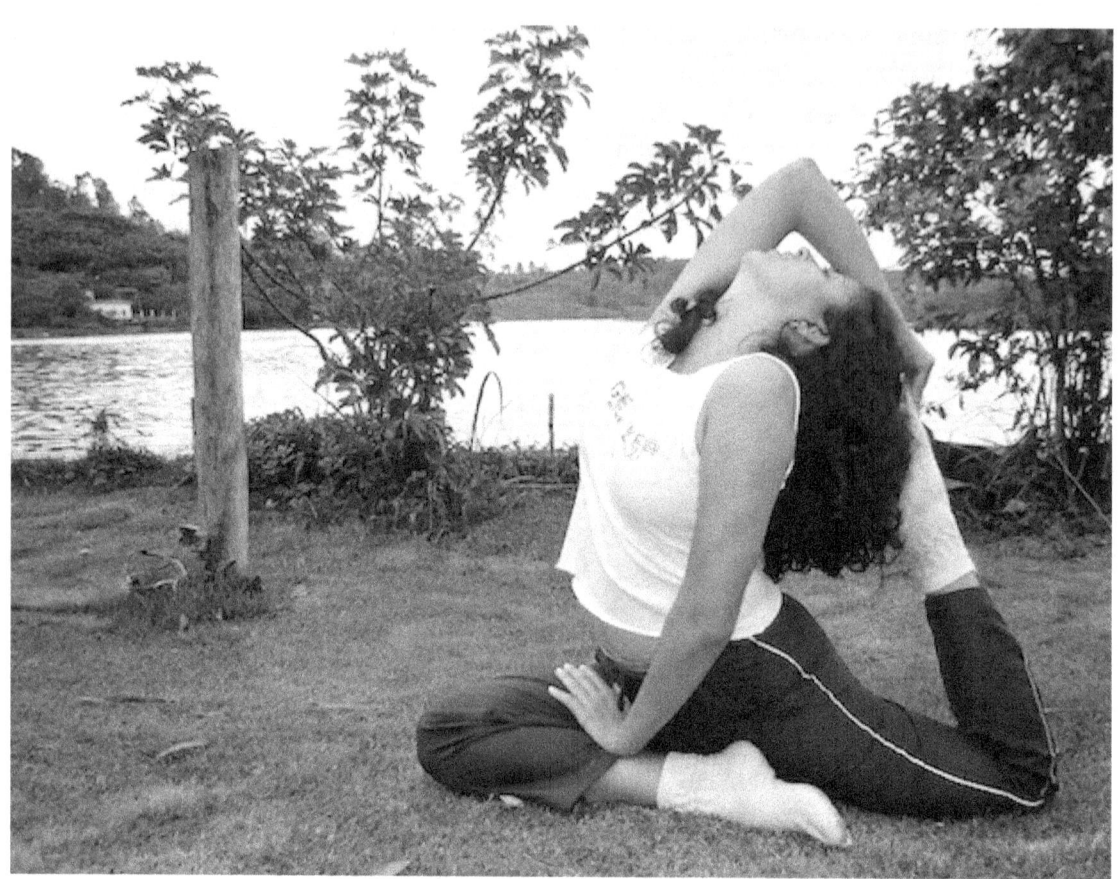

4. **Body Measurements/BMI/Weight Log:** This is important. Many people become discouraged early on in dieting because they don't see much weight difference on their scales. Many even gain weight. This is normal. At first, you may gain more muscle which can increase your weight on the scale. I always recommend that clients ditch the scale and only weigh in once per month. Instead, I encourage them to track their progress through body measurements. Even if weight is holding steady or increasing on the scales, you will find that body measurements are decreasing! If you weigh yourself once per week, you probably won't see much change, which can be very discouraging. But, if you take your body measurements once per week, you will see quite a bit of change, which can be oh so inspiring! This section will also be used to track your BMI - Body Mass Index (we will discuss how to measure and track both in few sections) as well as your monthly weigh-in Log. Here are some easy ways to set up this section:

First, a sample of an easy body measurements log:

Body Measurements Log						
Month/Year: January 2013						
		Week 1	Week 2	Week 3	Week 4	Week 5
NECK	Around largest part of the neck; directly across Adam's apple.	14¾"				
BUST	Measure all the way around your bust/back right at the nipple line. The tape should lay flat across the skin, not pressing in.					
CHEST	Measure under your breasts, as high up as the tape will go. Keep the tape in a straight line as you bring it around your back.					
UPPER ARMS	Measure wherever biggest ABOVE the elbows. (Write one measurement for each upper arm).					
FOREARMS	Measure wherever biggest BELOW the elbows. (Write one measurement for each forearm).					
WAIST	Your "natural waist" can be found 2-inches above your hip bone or at the smallest point between your breastbone and your belly button. Measure all the way around.					
ABS	Measure all the way around by placing tape directly over belly button.					
HIPS	When standing, press legs together and measure at the widest point of the buttocks, bring the tape all the way around.					
THIGHS	Spread your legs while standing; measure all the way around at the biggest part of your thigh. (Write one measurement for each thigh).					
CALVES	Measure all the way around wherever biggest. (Write one measurement for each of your calves).					

Next, a sample of an easy BMI log:

BMI (Body Mass Index) Log													
Year:2013													
	JAN	**FEB**	**MAR**	**APR**	**MAY**	**JUN**	**JUL**	**AUG**	**SEP**	**OCT**	**NOV**	**DEC**	
BMI	EXA MPLE 21.9												

AND finally, a sample of a fantastic weight loss log:

Monthly Weight Loss Log			
DATE	**WEIGHT**	**+/-**	**COMMENTS**
01/10/2013	148	-6	I am going for double that amount next month!
02/12/2013	140	-8	Oh, so close..!!!
03/11/2013	142	+2	Ooops! I will lose it again!

5. **Thoughts/Feelings:** This is the writing part of your journal. This is the area where you write whatever you want – concerns, fears, hopes, happy moments, and anything else that comes to min. Because this is the most intimate part of your journal, most people prefer to put it in the back as the last section.

Bonus Section (Optional): If you can find a 6-subject or more notebook or if you want to split up one of your five sections, here is an optional section title that you may want as a part of your journal. Note: This section, again, is optional only. The above sections are necessary.

6. **Recipes for Fasting:** As you become a pro at fasting and breaking up your fasting calories, you will begin researching and creating different low-calorie recipe ideas. Many of my clients adore their recipe section because as meal or ingredient ideas pop up in their minds (and they will in your mind too), they love having a place to unload those ideas.

Way to go! With your new weight loss journal by your side, you will have everything you need to be successful and inspired in one place. Many people who have reached their goal weight and kept a journal along the way swear that a large part of their success is credited to their weight loss journals. A weight loss journal will hold you accountable and it will keep you honest with yourself. When trying to lose weight, honesty and accountability are CRUCIAL.

Your First Fast

When preparing for your first fast there are some things you can do to make the fast easier and to make sure you are getting the most out of your first fast.

As your first fast approaches, you may become a bit nervous. You may be a little anxious, hoping that all goes well during the fast and worrying about whether or not you have it in you to complete the fast successfully. It is absolutely normal to be a little apprehensive about your first fast after all, you are about to venture into unknown territory and that can be nerve-wracking for anyone. Everyone remembers their very first fast, no matter if it lasted 10 hours or 10 days. They all remember how they felt right before, too. It is easy to be overwhelmed by the anticipation of wondering what will happen or how you'll feel along with the excitement of beginning a new adventure, a new journey, to a healthier and skinnier you! Here are some wonderful ideas and tips that will help your first fast be a successful and beneficial one:

Tip #1 - Plan ahead on how you will spread out your calories:

Okay, so you know that you are allowed a maximum of 500 calories per day for women and 600 calories for men (1/4 [25%] of your daily calorie intake). Let's say you are used to eating 2000 calories per day and then on the first day of your first fast, you knock your allowed 500 or 600 calories out on a big breakfast at 7:00 A.M. Now, for the rest of the day, you get to have nothing but water. How do you think you'd feel by 8:00 P.M. that same night? And, again, remember – this is the very first time you are experiencing what it is and how it feels to fast. Needless to say, by 8:00 P.M. you are probably moody, starving, and desperate.

Want to know how to prevent that nightmare situation from becoming a reality? Spread out those calories! There are many meals that are only 100 or 200 calories total – and, believe it or not, these super low-calorie meals are actually very filling and satisfying!

Let's focus on women for a minute. It is your first day of fasting. You have 24 hours and only 500 calories. Here is an excellent way to split those calories up:

Note: For the following meals and snacks mentioned, you can find the full recipe and nutritional data in the recipe section of this book.

Day One Fasting Schedule For a Woman	
7:00 P.M Night Before Fast	Finish your last meal BY 7:00 P.M. **FAST BEGINS NOW.**
7:00 A.M	**Wake-Up.** Great job! You are already 12 hours into your fast – only 12 hours to go!

9:00 A.M.	**Breakfast:** Tangy Mango Muffins (Serving Size: 1 muffin)	98 calories
11:00 P.M.	**Snack:** Breezy Watermelon Blast (Serving Size: 12-ounce glass)	33 calories
1:00 P.M.	**Lunch:** Spinach and Shrimp Salad (Serving Size: 1 salad)	59 calories
3:00 P.M	**Snack:** Chocolate Chip Cookies and ½ cup Skim Milk (Serving Size: 2 cookies)	110 calories
5:00 P.M.	**Dinner:** Greek Yogurt Topped Chickpea Veggie Burgers with Asian Cucumber Salad (Serving Size: 2 burgers & ½cup salad)	96 + 42 = 138 calories
Remember to account for calories from beverages and condiments if used!		
7:00 P.M.	**Fast is complete! Congratulations**	Total Calories: 466

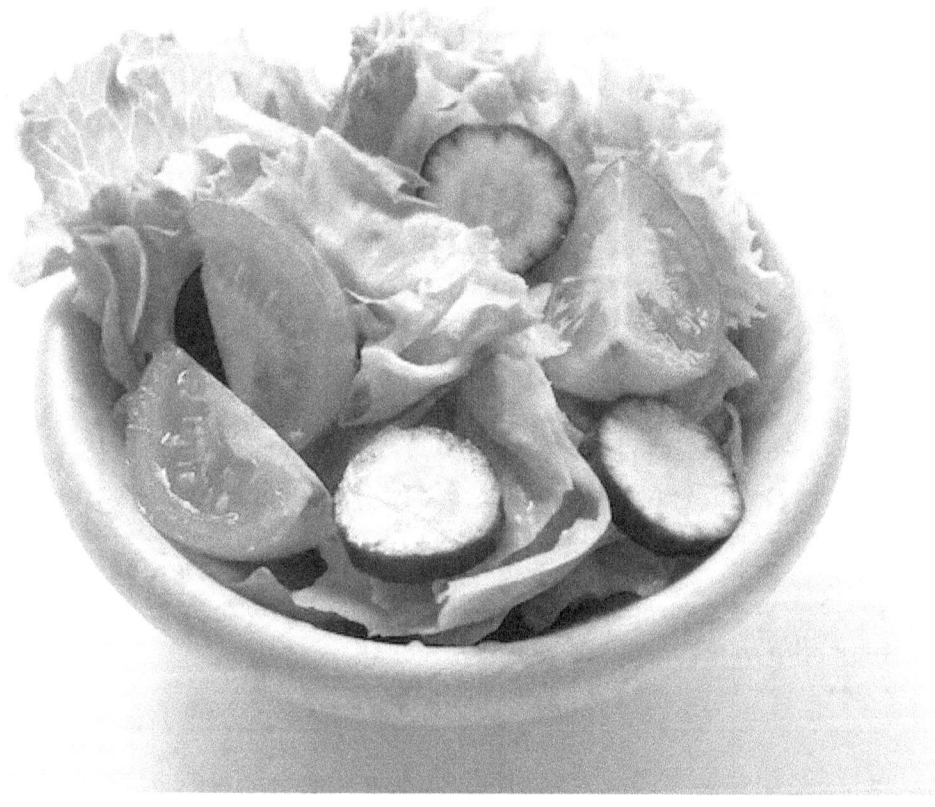

Can you believe you are able to do so much with so few calories? All of the recipes in this book, such as the ones above, are under 400 calories – most of them are under 200 calories. When you begin to figure out how to split up your fast-day calories on your own – just grab a calculator and flip through the recipes in the back of this book. By the time you make it through all of the recipes, you will be a pro at dividing up your fast calories and can start creating your own recipes if you'd like!

Tip #2 - Coffee is a MUST-HAVE for the Restricted Calorie Faster:

There is a popular mantra that intermittent fasters live by during their fasting cycles. It goes: **"Sidestep breakfast; opt for coffee instead, make lunchtime your first mealtime."** Because coffee is typically such a prominent part of fasting, many people worry that they will drop weight, but pick up a caffeine addiction. Yes, it is true that you can fall victim to a debilitating dependence on coffee – but, the way I see it – is that there are far worse things to which one could fall victim. In fact, there are a lot of great benefits from coffee:

- **Coffee accelerates fat burning and improves body composition**: When in a fasting state, coffee will mobilize your body fat so that your body burns it instead of glucose for energy. Coffee increases your metabolic rate so that you burn more calories faster, which means you attain a higher amount of weight lost faster!

- **Coffee helps suppress your appetite:** It will help you fight off hunger, which will help to keep you on track during your fast.

- **Coffee has protective properties and can reduce the risk of certain types of cancer:** Coffee fights many cancers, including lung, breast, stomach, prostate, colon, pancreatic, and endometrial cancers.

- **Coffee promotes vascular health:** Coffee helps to keep blood vessels healthy and improves vascular muscle tone. It also regulates blood pressure.

- **Coffee aids in cardiovascular health:** This drink significantly decreases the risk of heart disease and heart attacks.

- **Coffee reduces the risk of metabolic syndrome**: Drinking coffee daily lowers triglyceride levels and betters glucose tolerance.

- **Coffee reduces the risk of diabetes:** Coffee improves how quickly your body burns fat, influencing body composition, which can decrease your risk of diabetes.

- **Coffee improves cholesterol health:** The antioxidants in coffee have been shown to improve "bad" LDL cholesterol and raise "good" HDL cholesterol.

- **Coffee improves power and strength performance:** Drink a coffee before an intense workout. Rather than acting directly on the nervous system to produce greater power/strength, the caffeine in the coffee will instead act directly on the muscles themselves.

- **Coffee speeds recovery and relieves muscle soreness:** Drink coffee to help your body and muscle groups recover after a hard, powerful workout.

- **Coffee increases motivation and reaction time:** Coffee is known to make you more alert, and more able to focus. It also helps to motivate you – which is often needed during fasting!

Can you believe that so much power can be in one cup of coffee? Drink coffee to help you through your fasting and exercise! For those who do not like drinking coffee – I encourage you to do your best to try to drink it anyways. It is worth it for all of the amazing benefits.

By the way, when I say **coffee**, I am NOT referring to a 35,000 calorie *Venti-vanilla soy-quad shot-decaf-no foam-extra hot- peppermint white chocolate mocha, with whip and extra syrup* from Starbucks. I am referring to a cup of black coffee with, at the most, a splash of whole milk or soy milk and a pinch of Splenda. If you are wondering why I don't recommend non-fat, or even 2% milk, its because whole milk drinkers actually weigh less in the long run. Whole milk contains a fat fighting enzyme that reduced fat and non-fat milks do not contain – but that is the topic of an entirely different book!

Tip #3 - Keep Hydrated:

Water is more important than ever during a fast. You must keep yourself hydrated while fasting or you could get headaches, cramps, and just feel lousy overall. Water works wonders for those fasting – for one, it will keep you full! I always recommend that before you eat your fasting meals or snacks, you sit down and drink an 8-ounce glass of water. Wait 10 minutes, then eat. This will help your stomach feel fuller faster, which will help you feel satisfied.

During your fasting days, you will want to drink at least one gallon of water per fasting day. The more active you are, the more water you'll need during a fast. So, if you work out 3 hours per day, 5 days per week – you will need to drink closer to two gallons of water or more during your fasting cycles.

Tip #4 – Meals before Fasting:

Many people think that if they eat a huge meal for their last feed day meal, that they will be able to make it through their fast easier. Not true. In fact, eating a huge meal right before switching over to a fast day will only make you hungrier. Instead, choose a lighter meal that is focused on carbohydrates, some protein, and the use of oils and fats. They will delay the emptying of your stomach – which will make you feel fuller much longer than if you were to eat an enormous meal. Fruit is fine to eat with your pre-fast meal; because of the water content the fruit is digested bit by bit over a lengthy amount of time, making it so you feel satisfied longer after eating it. However, for your last pre-fast meal, avoid salad and high-fiber foods as they digest very quickly.

For your first feed day meals following each fast cycle, always eat a lighter meal with at least some type of fruit. This will ease your body back into your feed day calorie load, without making you sick to your stomach.

Tip # 5 – Wear loose, light, and comfortable clothing during your fast:

Do not wear anything too heavy or tight that could make you perspire. When you sweat, you lose water that your body desperately needs during your fasting cycle.

Tip # 6 – Take short naps during your fast if you are able:

This will help you to pass the time, and it's proven that people have a feeling of fullness and satisfaction following a short nap.

Tip # 7 – Sniff spices to satisfy feelings of hunger:

It may sound crazy, but this little trick works! If you begin craving foods or feeling hungry, high tail it to the spice cabinet and take in a couple whiffs of a pleasant spelling spice - then watch as your hunger floats away!

Tip # 8 – Organize your fast day recipes by calorie amounts:

When you organize all of your recipes according to calorie amount, you can easily plan your fast day meals by mixing and matching recipes. This is a great way to be able to add variety to each fast day.

When and What to Eat

Let's first talk about WHEN to eat:

You will find that your fast days become more about WHEN you eat rather than WHAT you eat. You want the 5:2 Diet to fit into your normal lifestyle and daily routine as smoothly and comfortably as possible.

First, it is important to pick the best fast/feed days for YOU! If you are reading an intermittent fasting book and the author fasts on Tuesday and Thursday, don't choose to do those days as well just because the author does it. If you choose Tuesdays/Thursdays to fast, it should be because those are the easiest days in your schedule for you to fast.

Let's say you and a close friend are doing the 5:2 Diet together. This is where it can get a little tricky. Of course, it would be ideal if your best days to feed/fast were the same as your friends – it would be a perfect way for the two of you to support and relate to each other's experiences. However, in the real world, things don't always work out the way they should. If your friend needs to fast on Monday and Wednesday, because those are her days off work, but you need to fast on Tuesday and Friday – stick with what best serves your own needs. Do not bend to accommodate someone else's style, and never feel guilty for not doing so. This is *your* journey.

You want to pick fast/feed days that accommodate your schedule best. When you choose your two fast days, you will need to consider several factors such as work, family obligations, lifestyle, and social commitments.

While you want to make the fast days as convenient for you as possible, you do not want to make it so your diet makes others miserable. For instance, let's say, this upcoming Tuesday your daughter wanted you to take her to a Mommy and daughter cookie baking class – but Tuesday happens to be a fast day and you know that your daughter and you will be eating the cookies as fast as you can bake them.

What to do? What to do?

Change your fast/feed days for next week! Remember: You can always change the days you feed and fast, every week if need be. As long as no two fast days are back-to-back, then you're golden. In fact, you will actually burn more fat and calories by mixing your days up – it's best to keep your body guessing. That will keep your metabolism running like mad! It's when you fall into a routine that your body adjusts to it and your metabolism slows. Never be afraid rearrange your fast/feed cycles – as a matter of fact, I recommend it.

Many 5:2 Diet participants opt for Mondays and Wednesdays for fasting. They have the weekend to eat well and usually prefer to eat lighter on Monday. Wednesday is great because it is still early enough in the week so that you can change your fast day to Thursday or Friday if need be, without it impacting any planned social events over the weekend.

One other important tip: only grocery shop on feed days. You don't want to find yourself in the middle of a fast day with a whole fresh stock of yummy foods in the fridge and pantry. Not fun..or fair!

As far as best times to eat – this is a bit harder to determine as it tends to vary from person to person. The plan is 500 calories for women, 600 calories for men – how to split those up has long been debated. Is it better to have one 500 or 600 calorie meal halfway through your fast day? Would you do better splitting it into two meals (breakfast and dinner) or three meals (breakfast, lunch, and dinner) or five small snacks?

The answer is that you should eat whenever it works best for you. It's better if you try to go as long as you can before eating. For example, if you typically eat lunch at 12:00 noon on your feed days, then try and push lunchtime to 2:00 or 3:00 P.M. on your fast days. It may take a few weeks and some experimenting to decide what works best for you, but when you finally find a protocol that gets you through your fast days with as few issues as possible, stick with it!

Now, let's discuss WHAT to eat:

As far as the best types of foods to eat during your fast days, you will want to eat foods that are packed with essential nutrients and vitamins. You want foods that are filling and slow to digest. Eat foods that are high in oils and fats as they will slow down the emptying of your stomach.

You will want to eat foods that are high in carbs and a little protein – avoid foods that are high in fiber as they will digest very quickly.

Eat lots of fruit - the water content helps you to feel full and satisfied for quite some time. Avoid salads and greens as they digest quickly and are not as satisfying or filling as is needed during your fasting cycle.

Drink lots and lots of water. Drink at least one gallon of water per fast day, and closer to two gallons if you are very active. Here is an excellent way to divide up your water throughout your fast day: Drink (1) 8-ounce glass before your meal(s)→ wait 10-minutes → Eat → Drink one more 8-ounce glass of water when finished with your meal. This protocol will keep you feeling satisfied for a significant amount of time. As far as beverages, you may drink:

- All the water you want.
- Coffee, black (hot and iced both acceptable)
- Teas (hot and cold both acceptable)
- Juice (100% Fruit or Vegetable – watch sugar content)
- Green smoothies and raw juices

Remember, you must also count the calories of any beverages you consume! People often only count the food calories and forget about the drink calories – this will throw you way off course!

To wrap up, when it comes to deciding *what* and *when* to eat, just use your best judgment. If it's a fast day, you know you only have 500/600 calories – so it's probably best not to wake up at 7:00A.M. and knock out your total allowed calories by downing two Snickers and a Mountain Dew by 7:15A.M. Eat smart, spread your calories out, and eat foods that are slow to digest and very filling. After a couple of months, you will be a pro at 5:2!

5:2 Diet and Optimum Health

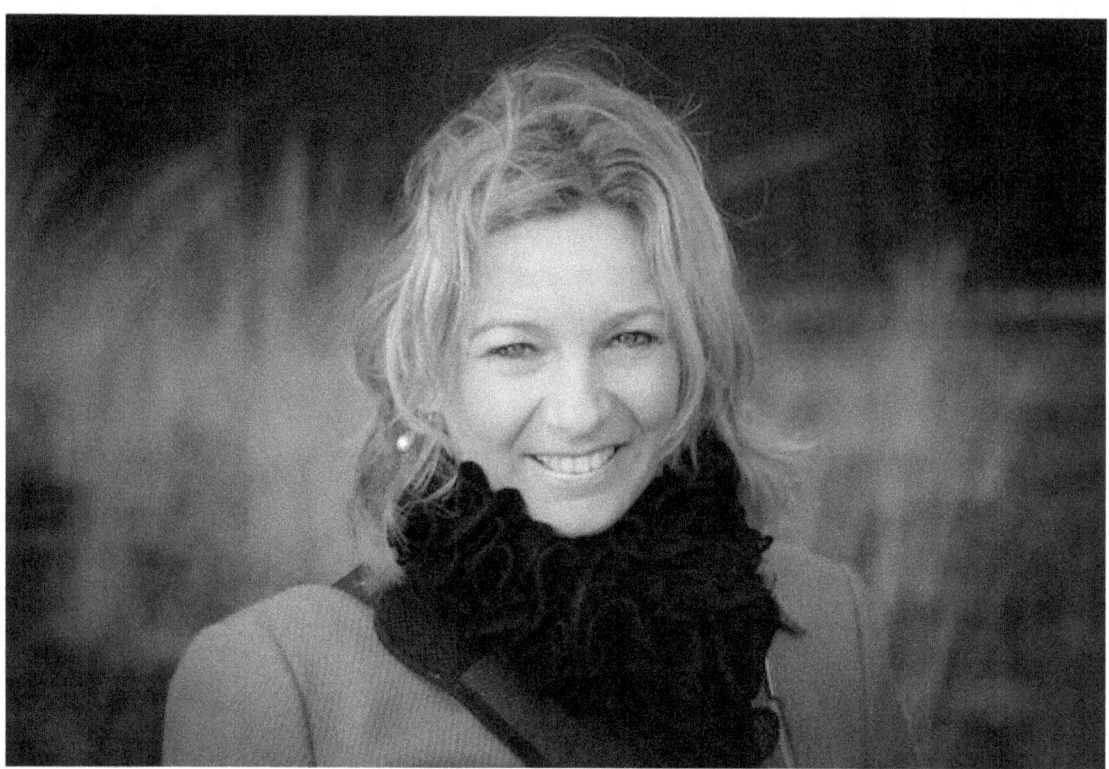

The 5:2 Diet does many things and offers many benefits. We mentioned many of them early on, but it is important enough topic to discuss in more detail. The most important benefit of 5:2 for many is, of course, the potential for weight loss. The possibility of losing weight is typically the leading force that first drives people toward the diet, but in all actuality, the 5:2 Diet is *so* much more than just a method of losing weight.

This diet has been scientifically proven to help you live longer, look younger, and feel better! It has been shown to reduce/reverse signs of aging and accelerated aging.

The 5:2 Diet promotes brain health. It has proven to support short- and long-term memory; it increases alertness and focus; it decreases the risk of brain diseases and disorders such as Alzheimer's, Dementia, and Parkinson's.

The 5:2 Diet is said to reverse metabolic syndrome in overweight women, as well as correct other metabolic issues. The fasting/feeding cycle speeds up the metabolic rate and pushes even the slowest metabolism into extreme fat burning mode. This diet has also proven to work successfully for those with thyroid conditions, when no other diets have had positive results!

The 5:2 Diet promotes many health benefits, both short- and long-term. It prevents many age-related diseases, it cures many ailments, and it reduces the severity of symptoms related to illness.

5:2 offers you a lifestyle that allows you to eat as you'd like 5 out of 7 days per week! Because you have the bulk of the week to eat as you wish, the risk of cheating, cravings, and binge eating decrease significantly. Sure, the fasts can be difficult at first as your body is attempting to adjust to the new eating schedule, however, any cravings you may have in the beginning will become less and less noticeable.

The 5:2 Diet promotes insulin and blood sugar balance. The diet lowers insulin levels which increases the rate at which your body burns fat, on top of that, when you do cardio during your fasting cycle, you will double to triple the amount of fat and calories burned. Many people think that they will be too tired or weak during their fast days to exercise, but after your first few fasts you will begin to find that you actually have more energy and are able to work out more intensely during fasting cycles. You are literally a fat and calorie-burning machine during your fast days!

Additionally, the 5:2 Diet, promotes organ health (particularly cardiovascular health), reduces blood pressure, cholesterol, glucose levels, repairs cells and genes, reduces inflammation, reduces blood lipids, and regulates bodily functions. The diet also detoxifies and cleanses the body.

This is a diet that gives you freedom and options – YOU choose your feeding/fasting cycle schedule. YOU choose which days of the week you want to feed/fast. YOU design the diet to fit around YOUR lifestyle – The 5:2 Diet finally gives you a diet that schedules itself around your life – no longer do you have to adjust your schedule to meet the demands of a diet. YOU are in charge – which is precisely the way it should be!

Maintaining a Healthy BMI (Body Mass Index)

Your BMI (Body Mass Index) is a great way to measure the amount of fat in your body through your height and weight. You can use your BMI to find out where your body fat falls according to your height and weight (underweight, normal weight, overweight, obese). The beauty of BMI, is that it can help you pinpoint how at risk you are for weight-related diseases within a matter of seconds. If your BMI says you are underweight, overweight or obese, then you know that your health is in jeopardy and that it is up to you to eat healthier, exercise, and to take better care of yourself until you are no longer in those danger zones.

I find it is much better to track your weight loss through body measurements and BMI than regular weight checks. Your weight on a scale is not always the greatest or most precise measurement of where you are in your journey. Sure, it can show you how much of a difference you have made thus far, but it can never show you the big picture. Only BMI and body measurements can. One week your weight on the scales may be exactly the same as the week before, but your body measurements have most likely decreased from the previous week's measurements. When losing weight, you want to have the most accurate view of your progress. While it is important to check your weight each month, you should also complete weekly body measurements and monthly BMI calculations.

Another factor to consider about BMI is that the difference between underweight to normal weight; normal weight to overweight; and overweight to obese can be as little as one pound. For each category there is a weight range. A person can lose and gain weight daily depending on the amount of water they consume, how much they eat, as well as the last time they ate or went to the bathroom. Therefore, the best time to check your BMI is when you first wake up, before you eat, drink, or use the restroom – this will give you the most accurate reading.

Finding out one's BMI is really nothing more than understanding a math equation. People tend to make understanding one's BMI more complicated than it needs to be. The formula is simple really:

Imperial BMI Formula

To begin, your height in inches needs to be squared (for a quick math term refresher, "squared" means to the 2nd power so if you are 72 inches tall, you would multiply 72 x 72 = 5184. 5184 is 72 inches squared, or 72 inches^2)Remember, always square your height in inches first! Next, multiply your weight in pounds by 703 (This number is needed because BMI was originally calculated using the metric system so in order for the imperial calculations to be precise, this is the number that you will always multiply your weight in pounds by. It will never change). Finally, take that number and divide it by your height^2. For example:

Sue weighs 155lbs. and is 67 inches tall. To find her BMI, use the following formula (Note: h = height; w= weight):

$$BMI = w(703)/h^2$$

Let's work out that formula:

(X = BMI)
67 inches^2 (67 x 67 = 4489)
155lbs x 703 = 108,965
108,965/4489 = 24.27 (round to the second decimal point)

X = 24 (Sue's BMI is 24)

Metric BMI Formula

The BMI was originally calculated using the metric system and this is still the way many people prefer to determine BMI. To find your BMI using metric calculations you divide your weight in kilograms by your height in meters squared. Use the following formula (Remember: w = weight; h = height):

$$BMI = w/h^2$$

Let's use the same example as before -

Sue weighs 70kg.s and is 1.7m tall. To find her BMI, use the following formula (Note: h = height; w= weight):

BMI = X

$1.7^2 = 2.89$

70/2.89 = 24.22 (Round to the second decimal point)

X = 24 (Sue's BMI is, again, 24)

Now you try calculating your own BMI, using either the Imperial or Metric methods:

Imperial BMI Formula

Name: _____	Date: _____

| Height (inches) _____ | |
| Weight (pounds) _____ | |

First, calculate your height in inches squared h^2	_____ (answer #1)
Next, multiply your weight in pounds by 703	_____ (answer #2)
Now, divide answer #2 by answer #1 to get answer #3	_____ (answer #3)
Finally, round answer #3 to second decimal point, for your total BMI	_____ (My BMI)

Metric BMI Formula

Name: _____	Date: _____

| Height (kilograms) _____ | |
| Weight (meters) _____ | |

First, calculate your height in meters squared h^2	_____ (answer #1)
Next, divide your weight in kilograms by answer #1 to get answer #2	_____ (answer #2)
Round answer #2 to second decimal point for Total BMI	_____ (My BMI)

Great job! Once you understand how to determine your BMI, you will find that it is a wonderful tool in tracking your progress. Use the chart below to see if you calculated correctly. It is for informational purposes only when attempting to understand BMI.

Note: Weight has been rounded off in the chart. If you cannot find your height/weight in the chart, know that you will be able to in a standard chart.

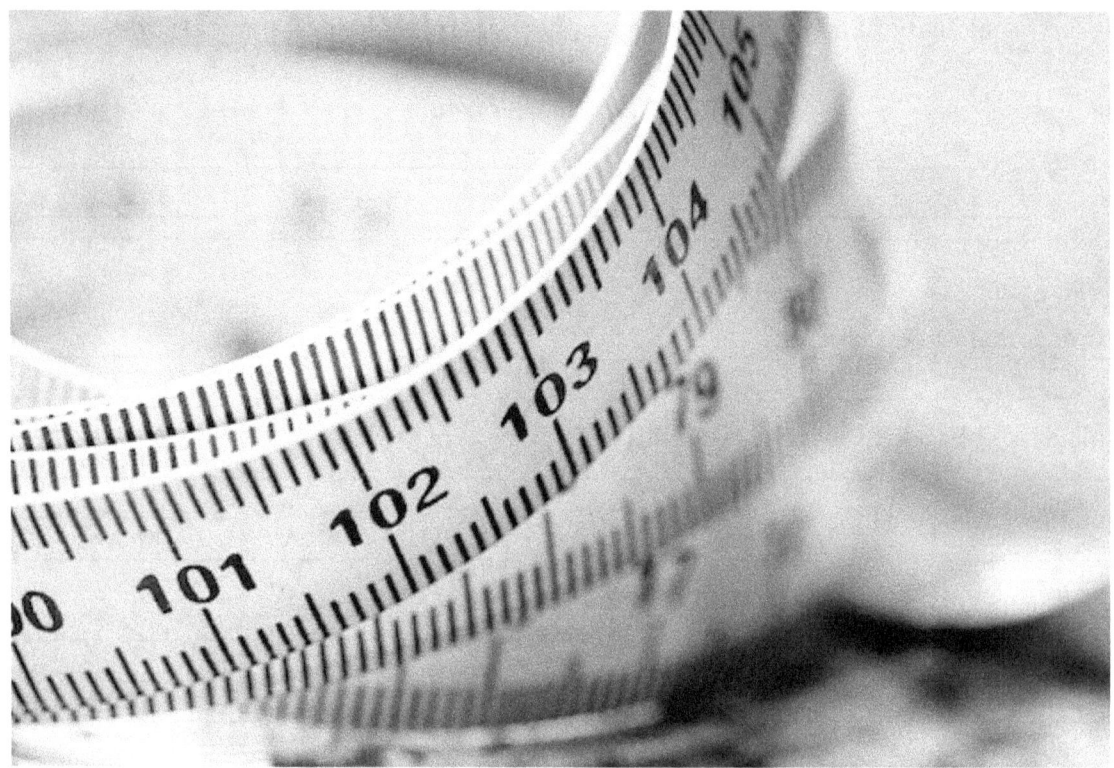

BMI (BODY MASS INDEX) CHART																	
BMI	**19**	**20**	**21**	**22**	**23**	**24**	**25**	**26**	**27**	**28**	**29**	**30**	**31**	**32**	**33**	**34**	**35**
Height (In.)	**Body Weight (Pounds)**																
58	91	96	100	105	110	115	119	124	129	134	138	143	148	153	158	162	167
59	94	99	104	109	114	119	124	128	133	138	143	148	153	158	163	168	173
60	97	102	107	112	118	123	128	133	138	143	148	153	158	163	168	174	179
61	100	106	111	116	122	127	132	137	143	148	153	158	164	169	174	180	185
62	104	109	115	120	126	131	136	142	147	153	158	164	169	175	180	186	191
63	107	113	118	124	130	135	141	146	152	158	163	169	175	180	186	191	197
64	110	116	122	128	134	140	145	151	157	163	169	174	180	186	192	197	204
65	114	120	126	132	138	144	150	156	162	168	174	180	186	192	198	204	210
66	118	124	130	136	142	148	155	161	167	173	179	186	192	198	204	210	216
67	121	127	134	140	146	153	159	166	172	178	185	191	198	204	211	217	223
68	125	131	138	144	151	158	164	171	177	184	190	197	203	210	216	223	230
69	128	135	142	149	155	162	169	176	182	189	196	203	209	216	223	230	236
70	132	139	146	153	160	167	174	181	188	195	202	209	216	222	229	236	243
71	136	143	150	157	165	172	179	186	193	200	208	215	222	229	236	243	250
72	140	147	154	162	169	177	184	191	199	206	213	221	228	235	242	250	258
73	144	151	159	166	174	182	189	197	204	212	219	227	235	242	250	257	265
74	148	155	163	171	179	186	194	202	210	218	225	233	241	249	256	264	272
75	152	160	168	176	184	192	200	208	216	224	232	240	248	256	264	272	279
76	156	164	172	180	189	197	205	213	221	230	238	246	254	263	271	279	287

Understanding BMI Charts and Results

This whole BMI thing may seem a bit tricky at first, but once you get the hang of it, you will realize how simple the process truly is. A standard BMI chart is the same for men, women, and teens. There are special BMI charts available for children since their bodies are so different in size from that of a teenager or adult.

A standard BMI chart follows a good height/weight range to meet the data of most individuals. If you are exceptionally tall or short, or weigh more or less than the weight range on standard BMI charts, there are BMI charts available out there to meet your height/weight needs. Try researching BMI charts online until you find a chart that meets your needs. You can also print out or purchase these charts so that you can keep them in your 5:2 Diet journal. Note: The chart above is, again, just a sample chart. Most standard BMI charts have more of a height/weight range.

Let's look at the categories that your BMI can fall into:

Keep in mind, that different agencies and nations may use different ranges on their BMI charts to determine weight class. The below categories and weight ranges are in accordance with the U.S. Department of Health and Human Services – which, for Americans, is the best BMI classification system to use.

BMI Standard Weight Classes	
Below 18.5	Underweight
18.5 to 24.9	Normal Weight
25 to 29.9	Overweight
30 and Above	Obese

Remember, the best time to check your BMI is first thing in the morning on an empty stomach, before you use the restroom. Check your BMI at least once per month to keep track of your weight loss progress!

Exercising on the 5:2 Diet

As we've already discussed, exercise and fasting are a dieter's secret weapons. It has been scientifically proven that exercising on an empty stomach offers more health and fitness benefits and keeps you young. Literally - there is evidence that exercising while fasting will reverse or prevent biological aging! Many people have had their ears filled with all sorts of opinions and ideas about how, when, or if they should exercise while fasting. Everyone is an expert, right? Well, for the moment, I want you to forget all you know or have heard about intermittent fasting and exercise. I want you to read the following information with a clear and open mind.

First, let's talk science. You may have heard of your Sympathetic Nervous System, also referred to as SNS? The SNS is a part of your body's Autonomic Nervous System; it is the system that makes your body react to different stimuli. It delivers that "fight or flight" response. It is what makes you react and respond to fear, excitement, danger, anticipation, motivation, or even sensations like pain or pleasure. For example, you know when you feel scared, you may get the chills or "goosebumps" up and down your arms? This is your SNS causing your body to respond to your fear. Your SNS will trigger your body to respond to different situations and stimuli in various ways:

- You can begin to sweat.
- Your pupils can dilate.

- Your heart rate can increase.
- The hair on your arms or the back of your neck may rise.
- You may be filled with an undeniable urge to flee.

There are many ways that your SNS can make your body react, and it is in charge of many bodily processes. What does this have to do with fasting and weight loss, you ask? Well, both exercising and fasting activate your SNS. This is beneficial to losing weight because your SNS is ALSO in charge of your body's fat burning process. So, when the exercising and fasting activate your SNS, your body naturally begins to burn fat like crazy!

Another piece of scientific proof that indicates exercise is more beneficial during fasting is the presence of HGH inside your body. HGH (Human Growth Hormone), also known as the "Fitness Hormone" is activated and the level of HGH in your body increases every time you exercise. High levels of HGH promote weight loss, and muscle growth. The hormone has anti-aging properties, it helps increase performance and endurance, it helps you stay naturally energized, and it rejuvenates you from the inside out. HGH is a miracle hormone to those trying to lose weight and through fasting and exercise; your levels of HGH will skyrocket naturally. Studies have shown that even higher levels of HGH are released when you are exercising while your body is in a fasting state. Research shows that fasting increases the levels of HGH by 1,200 to 1,400 percent in women and 1,800 to 2,000 percent in men!

There are many other reasons that support the fact that exercising while fasting will get you to your goal weight fast, you just have to try it out and see the difference for yourself. If you do not like exercising and can only force yourself to do it once or twice a week, then at least save your workouts for your fast days. Believe it or not, you can receive more benefits exercising on one day of fasting than you could on three days of feeding!

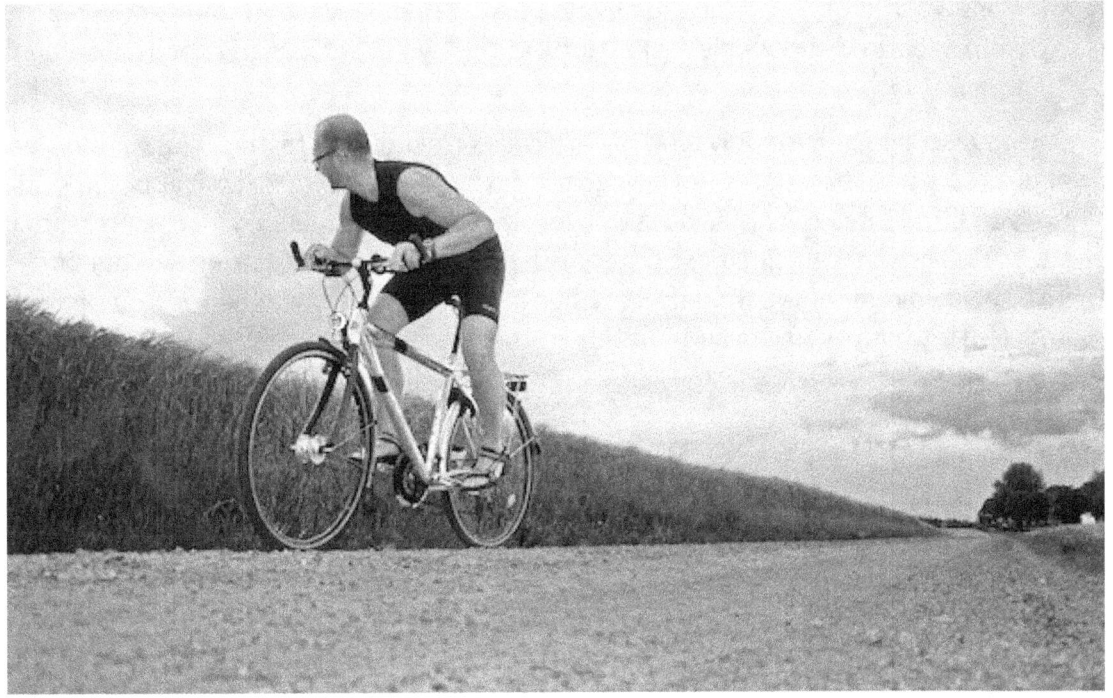

When and What Type of Exercise to do on Fast Days

There have been many debates over when to exercise and what type of exercise should be completed during a fasting cycle. The answer to WHEN is easy: The best time to exercise during fasting is first thing in the morning on a completely empty stomach, before you have eaten breakfast. As for WHAT type of exercising should be completed during fasting, that is entirely up to you. It depends on how you feel and what you can endure. When you first begin fasting, you should pick a fitness routine that you are comfortable with.

If you are new to exercise and to fasting, then start out slowly with light and short exercise intensity and duration. If you are already a gym rat but are new to fasting, bring your fitness intensity down a few notches at first. Your body will react differently to exercise when in a fasting state, so wait until you know how your body responds to fasting before kicking it back into high gear. If you are new to exercise but a pro at fasting, pick a fitness regimen that gets increasingly harder each week. You already know how your body feels and responds during fasting, so you can begin adjusting your fitness levels to a level at which your fasted body excels.

The idea here is to adopt a fitness regimen that is as intense as you are able to physically endure without overdoing it. Remember: the more intense the workout in a fasted state, the more fat and calories burned. If you haven't exercised a day in 20 years, but you decide to run 10 miles on the day of your very first fast you will only put yourself at risk for injuries, burnout, and more. Slow and steady wins the race. Once you become more familiar with your fasted body and you exercise regularly, you can begin to bump up the intensity and lengths of time you exercise.

You NEVER want your workout to be easy – there is no challenge in that and your body will not burn as many calories or fat if you do not have to exert yourself. On the other hand, you do not want your workouts to be so intense that you are injuring your body or unable to sit or stand for 3 days following a workout. You goal is to always be at a fitness level that falls somewhere in between comfortable and impossible. Take a look at the two best types of exercise for the fasted body:

- **Cardiovascular Exercise:** Any type of cardio is perfect during fasting. You should always plan to do some form of cardio during your fasting cycle. If you exercise regularly, aim for at 45 to 60 minutes of cardio, but set a goal for at least 30 minutes. Beginners, should start at 20 minutes and increase that time by 5 to 10 minutes each week. Your body an incredible amount of fat and calories when in a fasted state, so when you combine cardio and a fasted body, you can burn up three times more fat and calories! Different types of cardio workouts include:

  - Sprinting, Running, Jogging, Brisk Walking
  - Hiking, Mountain Biking, Skiing, Snowboarding
  - Step Aerobics, Spinning (Cycling), Kickboxing
  - Treadmill, Elliptical Machine, Stationary Bike, Rowing
  - Zumba, P90X, and other Home Based DVD Workouts
  - Swimming, Water Aerobics

- Sports (Soccer, Basketball, Football, Baseball, etc.)
- Trampolines, Stair Climbing, Wall Climbing, Jumping Rope, Dancing
- And many more..

- **Interval Training:** Try interval training for an intense workout. With interval training, you will burn quite a bit of fat. Interval training involves a mixture of low- and high-intensity cardio for a set amount of time. For example, on a treadmill interval training might look like this:

Total Interval Time: ___ minutes		
Incline	Speed	Minutes
2%	3.0mph	5
12%	2.5mph	2
4%	3.2mph	3
9%	4.8 mph	1
2%	3.0mph	5

- **Strength Training (Resistance Training):** Strength training is perfect for building muscle and toning your body. It focuses on working out specific muscles or muscle groups through repetitions.

  For beginners to intermediate fitness levels, it is best to do resistance training in 1 to 3 sets of 10 – 15 repetitions. Here is an example for those who are brand new to resistance training:

Resistance Training

Exercise: Bicep curls with 3lb. dumbbell

Sets: 3

Repetitions: 10

Beginning with either your left or right arm, begin set #1 by doing 10 bicep curls. Switch arms and do 10 bicep curls. You have just completed your first set.

Rest 15 to 30 seconds.

Begin Set #2 using the same arm you began set #1 with.

Rest 15 to 30 seconds.

Begin Set #3 using the same arm you began sets 1 & 2 with.

Finished.

For advanced fitness levels, you can do resistance training to the point of "failure" (the term "failure" refers to the point where you are unable to physically endure another set). Types of strength training include:

- **Weight/Resistance Machines**
- **Free Weights**
- **Calisthenics (Sit Ups, Crunches, Push Ups, Squats, Pull Ups, Dips, etc.)**
- **Resistance Bands**
- **Kettle Balls**
- **Medicine Balls**
- **Cable Resistance**
- **One's Own Body Weight**
- **Pilates/Yoga/Yogilates (a form of Yoga and Pilates rolled in one).**
- **Ankle, Wrist, and Other Wearable Training Weights**

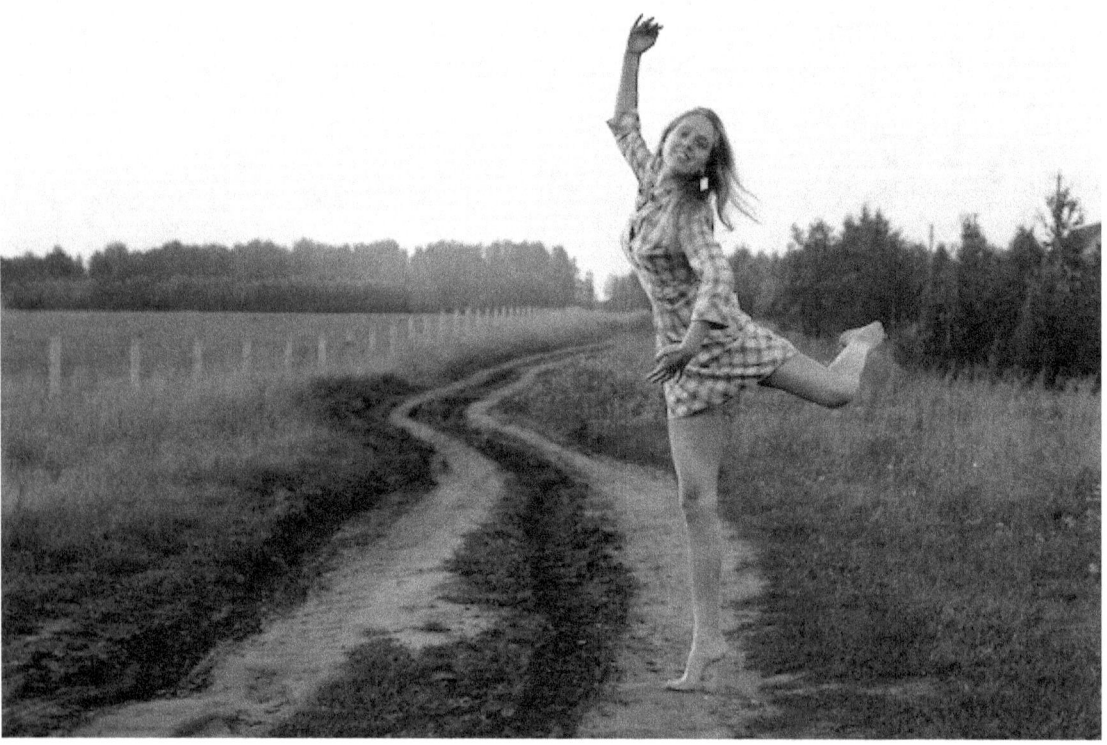

I believe that the secret to obtaining optimum results on 5:2 is to split up your workout on both fasting days. Let's say you are committing to a 60-minute workout on each fast day. Instead of doing one 60-minute workout, try this:

5:2 Week 1 Fast Day Fitness Regimen

Fast Day #1:

- When you wake up in the morning before you eat breakfast:
    - → Drink at least (1) 8-oz. of water (mandatory)
    - → Drink (1) 8-oz. cup of black coffee (optional)
    - → Complete 30-minutes worth of cardio (type of choice)
    - → Wait at least 15 to 30-minutes, then eat a light post-workout "recovery" meal with some carbs and a little protein.
- Eat NO MORE food after 2:00 P.M. (For your afternoon workout, you must not have eaten any food within 2 hours pre-workout).
- At 4:00 P.M.:
    - → Drink at least (1) 8-oz. of water (mandatory)
    - → Drink (1) 8-oz. cup of black coffee (optional)
    - → Complete 30-minutes worth of resistance training (type of choice)
    - → Wait at least 15 to 30-minutes, then eat post-workout "recovery" meal with some carbs and a little protein. This may be a larger meal than your first "recovery" meal.

Fast Day #2:

- Repeat same process as fast day #1, HOWEVER, switch cardio to afternoon workout and resistance training to morning workout.

The ideal scenario would be to dedicate yourself to (2) 45- to 60-minute workouts (1 cardio /1 resistance) on your fast days.

During your feed days, you can exercise as you like. You should give your body at least one day per week to rest - just NOT on a fast day, as this is when you will burn the most fat/calories. Starting out, try to aim for 20-30 minutes of exercise 3 to 5 days per week. Remember, to always workout on your fast days!

I realize many of you are anxious to get going and are motivated and excited about losing weight, but don't overdo it on exercising. Push your body; just don't push it to the point where it shuts down. You do not want to be laid-up for 3-weeks due to an injury that could have been prevented. Your body is a miraculous machine, but if you push it too hard, you will injure yourself. Again, for those who are already workout gurus, you already know how far you can push your bodies.

For those new to fitness, you need to take it in stages, listen to your body when you are working out and learn how your body reacts and responds to exercise. Rule of thumb: if you are breathing easy and have barely broken a sweat, you are taking it too easy and you need to bump up the intensity. On the other hand, if you are drenched in sweat, unable to catch your breath, and you feel like your heart is going to jump right out of your chest and take off running – then it is a safe bet that you are doing too much, too soon.

Target Heart Rate:

Monitoring your Target Heart Rate (THR) is one of the most beneficial ways to 1) ensure that you have reached the heart rate needed to burn the most fat and calories and 2) to determine if you are exercising safely.

You first need to learn how to determine your Maximum Heart Rate (MHR). According to the American Heart Association the best, and easiest, way to determine your MHR is to subtract your age from the number 220. For instance, if you are 35 years-old, your MHR would be 185. While working out you want to make sure that you do not exceed a heart rate of 185. Note: If you are taking any type of blood pressure or heart medications, you will want to consult your physician first, as the medication could affect the accuracy of determining your MHR. Additionally, keep in mind that your MHR will change slightly year by year as you age.

Once you know your MHR, you can then determine your Target Heart Rate (THR). First, you want to find your normal resting heart rate. A normal resting heart rate for adults is between 50-80 beats per minute, however 50-60 beats per minute is also considered normal. When exercising, you want to make sure that after warm-up, you reach your THR range and do your best to stay within that range throughout the rest of your workout. Always remember to cool down in order to bring you heart rate back to a normal level.

Note: The following chart can be used as a foundation to ensure that your heart rate calculations are accurate.

Target Heart Rate			
(Heart Beats Per Minute)			
Age	60%	80%	MHR (Beats/Min)
	Max	Max	
20	120	160	200
25	117	156	195
30	114	152	190
35	111	148	185
40	108	144	180
45	105	140	175
50	102	136	170
55	99	132	165
60	96	128	160
65	93	124	155
70	90	120	150

Let's examine the chart for a moment and look at an example.

Let's pretend you are 30 years-old. When you are exercising you need to maintain a target heart rate range between 114 and 152 beats per minute. You also must not exceed your MHR, which according to the chart (as well as the formula 220 - Age = MHR) is 190.

Easy enough right? However, it does get a bit tougher. Most charts, such as the one above, round ages out to the nearest 5th year. You will need to use the following formulas to find your EXACT Target Heart Range.

Lowest Target Heart Rate:
To find your lowest THR, use the following formula –
MHR x 60% (or .6) = Lowest THR

Let's use an example:
Greg is 38 years-old. First, we find his Maximum Heart Rate:
220 – 38 = 182 (MHR = 182)

Now, you take Greg's MHR of 182 and you multiply it by 60% or .6
$$182 \times 60\% \text{ (or .6)} = 109$$
Greg's Lowest Target Heart Rate is **109**.

Highest Target Heart Rate:
To find your highest THR, use the following formula –
$$\text{MHR} \times 80\% \text{ (or .8)} = \text{Highest THR}$$

Let's continue using Greg as an example:
Reminder: Greg is 38 years-old. His maximum heart rate (MHR) is **182**.
Now we can find his highest target heart rate. To do this, you take Greg's MHR of 182 and you multiply it by 80% or .8
$$182 \times 80\% \text{ (or .8)} = 145.5 \text{ (Round up to get 146)}$$
Greg's Lowest Target Heart Rate is **146**.

Let's determine now determine your target heart rate range. Complete the following activity to determine what your target heart rate range is for exercise.

My Heart Rate Zones:

Date:

Age:

Resting Heart Rate (RHR): _____
To find your RHR sit down for at least five minutes. Then take your pulse while watching a clock and count each beat for 15 seconds. When finished, take the number of beats you counted and multiply that number by 4. The result will be your resting heart rate. Note: Your RHR many change each and every time you check it – this is natural, just make sure that it always falls within the normal range for adults which is 60 to 80 beats per minute, but may be as low as 50.

Maximum Heart Rate (MHR): _____
Now let's find your MHR. Remember the formula?
220 – _____(Your Age) = _____ MHR). Use this formula to calculate your MHR. Take the number 220 and subtract your age. The resulting number is your MHR.

Target Heart Rate (THR) Range: Lowest THR_____   Highest THR_____
To find your THR, all you need is your age and the chart on the following page and a few calculations. Your target heart rate range is broken up into three different zones for exercise. The zones help you to determine the amount of effort you are exerting during your workout. The higher the zone, the more fat and calories you are burning:

Lowest THR: MHR x 60% (or .6) = _____
Highest THR: MHR x 80% (or .8)= _____

- **Zone 1: 60% - Lower Range of THR**
- **Zone 2: 80% - Higher Range of THR**
- **Zone 3: 100% - Your MHR (Do not Exceed)**

Once you have all of this information, you have everything you need to exercise safely and effectively while on the 5:2 Diet. For optimum results, remember to check your heart rate regularly while exercising. Make sure you are always within your THR range and not exceeding your MHR.

Note: The following chart can be used as a foundation to ensure that your heart rate calculations are accurate.

Target Heart Rate			
(Heart Beats Per Minute)			
Age	60%	80%	MHR (Beats/Min)
	Max	Max	
20	120	160	200
25	117	156	195
30	114	152	190
35	111	148	185
40	108	144	180
45	105	140	175
50	102	136	170
55	99	132	165
60	96	128	160
65	93	124	155
70	90	120	150

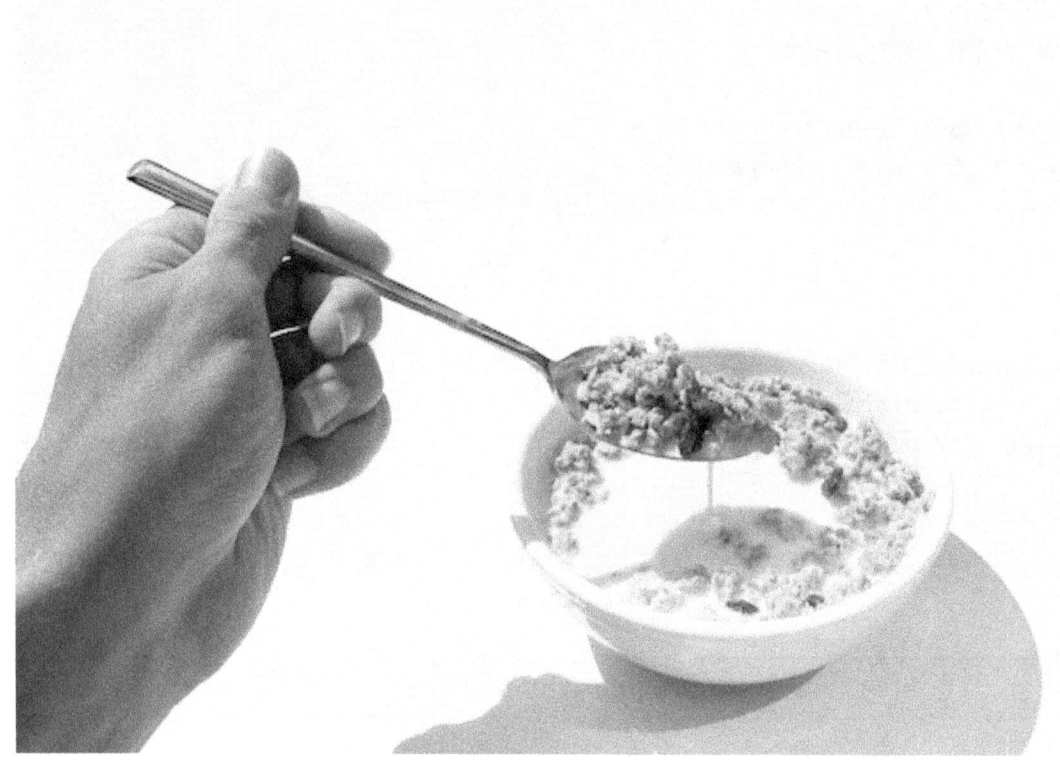

5:2 Diet/Intermittent Fasting FAQ's

Listed below are some of the most common questions people have concerning the 5:2 Diet and/or intermittent fasting.

Q: What is the 5:2 Diet in a one-sentence summary?

A: The 5:2 Diet is a combination of weekly cycles of 2-day severe low-calorie fasting and 5-day normal feeding to trick the body into action, in order to gain ultimate weight loss, optimum health, and increased vitality.

Q: Is the 5:2 Diet flexible?

A: The 5:2 Diet is absolutely flexible and very convenient. Finally, a diet that fits around you and your lifestyle! You can change up the days you fast or feed, you can mix up your daily calorie intake as long as you are not exceeding 2000 calories for women/2400 calories for men on feed days, and as long as your fast days do not exceed 25% of your daily feed calories. You also have the option of changing the amount of fast or feed days each week. For example, instead of 5:2 (5 days feeding/2 days fasting) you could try 4:3 (4 days feeding/3 days fasting). You just need to make sure that the fast days are non-consecutive.

Q: Isn't "fasting" supposed to mean NO food?

A: There are different types of fasting. On 5:2, the idea is for you to be able to "fast" in a way that gives you all of the health and weight loss benefits of fasting without the trouble of NO food. It has been shown that more people will stick to an intermittent fasting diet, like 5:2, because even though they are allowed little to eat on fast days, they are still able to eat, and that gives them the motivation to stick with it. You do have the option to complete water or juice fasts - this is a fast where you consume only water and/or juice - on your fast days, and many people on 5:2 will opt to complete a no-food fast on one of their fast days in order to really rejuvenate and re-group. There is nothing more beneficial for your body, besides water, than the occasional no-food fast.

You always have a choice to complete a no-food fast, but for the sake of really sticking with the 5:2 Diet, it is important that you understand that while you can do a no-food fast, you are not obligated to do so.

Q: How much weight can I expect to lose on the 5:2 Diet?

A: As with anything, results vary from person to person. It depends on how dedicated you are to the 5:2 regimen as well as how long you plan to participate in 5:2. Ask anyone who has been on the 5:2 Diet for over 4 months, and they will tell you that if you work the diet like you are supposed to, you can easily meet your weight loss goals. How much weight you lose also depends on the amount of exercise you are combining with the diet. Studies have shown that 5:2 dieters who workout at least three days per week, with two of those days being fast days, will lose weight at a faster rate than 5:2 dieters who workout on three of the feed days. Remember, your best bet for optimum results is to exercise on your fast days, as you burn more and burn faster.

The sky is the limit with 5:2. It doesn't matter if you set a weight loss goal of 5lbs., 50lbs., or 500lbs. If you work the diet as you are supposed to, 5:2 will get you to your goals – whatever they are!

Q: Will fasting make me feel ill?

A: 5:2 should not make you feel sick to your stomach or result in any unpleasant side effects, because you are still feeding your body, even on fast days. This being said, every person is different and therefore reacts differently to 5:2. In my years of experience helping guide people through their 5:2 journeys, I have come to expect that if any 5:2 participants begin to feel ill or presents with minor adverse side effects, it is almost always in the very beginning, within their first few fasts. This is usually because their bodies are beginning to try to adapt to the new diet. If you begin to feel ill, either on a fast or feed day, don't become discouraged. Rest, sip on some tea, or ginger ale, and know that this unpleasant feeling will pass. Take solace in knowing that your body is working overtime to adjust to the diet so that you will receive optimum results.

If, for whatever reason, you are still feeling ill after a couple weeks of fasting, it would be best to consult your doctor to rule out anything serious.

Q: What can I eat during my fast days?

A: While fasting, you can eat anything you want as long as you do not exceed your maximum allowed calories, which are typically 500 calories for women and 600 calories for men. What you eat and when you eat it is up to you. You can eat one big 500/600 calorie meal or (2) 300/350 calories meals, or even several small snack throughout the day.

For beginners, it would be best for you to try and spread out your allowed calories as much as possible to avoid hunger, cravings, cheating, or binge eating as soon as you hit a feed day. Try to eat carbs and foods that are filling, satisfying, and slow to digest. Some foods, such as salad greens and high-fiber foods, digest easily and empty the stomach very quickly. Try to avoid these types of food while fasting. Fresh fruit is a wonderful choice. The water content in fruit will keep you feeling full for quite some time.

Q: Do I have to split up my two fast days?

A: Splitting the two fast days makes the 5:2 more manageable for some people. The goal of splitting the fast is to make the diet easy enough to stick with, while still ensuring that it is challenging your body. Your body will benefit and you will be able to achieve your health and weight goals following this plan.

Intermittent fasting dieters on programs such as 5:2 have proven successful in sticking with the diet overall when their fasting days are non-consecutive. Studies have shown that more people will stick with a fasting regimen that lasts 16 to 48 hours then they will with a fasting regimen that lasts longer than 48 hours. Fasting regimens that last longer than 48 hours have shown to put dieters at a much higher risk of cheating on their fasts, binge eating on feed days, and quitting the diet altogether. When first beginning 5:2 it is highly recommended that you stick with fasting on non-consecutive days.

If, after a few months, when you better understand 5:2 and you know how your mind and body responds to fasting, you decide you want to try putting your two fast days together; go for it! As a matter of fact, there are many 5:2 dieters who have found that 24 hour fasting is really easy for them, so they choose to put their fast days back-to-back for a 48 hour fast. This is great, because they can knock out their weekly fast days at once, and relax the rest of week. If you do decide to fast back-to-back, just make certain not to extend your fast beyond a 48 hour period.

The rule here is that you do whatever is most comfortable, and whatever works best for you. The main goal is to do whatever it takes to make you stick with 5:2.

Q: Can anyone participate in the 5:2 Diet?

A: As with any weight loss program it is best to consult with your doctor before beginning any diet regimen or program.

For the most part, 5:2 is a very safe diet. You are getting all the nutrition you need, you are not plaguing your body with weight loss pills that have yet to be approved by the FDA, you are not putting your bodies through any drastic or extreme measures. Pretty much anyone can safely participate in 5:2. Some exceptions are listed below, however.

The following groups should refrain from participating in intermittent fasting, since their conditions/situations call for a particular type of nutritional regimen, and dramatic diet changes could prove harmful. If one of the following areas refers to you, but you still would like to try 5:2, please consult your physician first. Your physician may be able to provide you with a safer way to participate in intermittent fasting, or a more appropriate alternative to meet your personal needs.

- Those who have type 1 or type 2 diabetes or are hypoglycemic should refrain from participating in 5:2.

- Those with autoimmune issues or those who are severely vitamin deficient should not participate in 5:2.

- Women who are pregnant, trying to become pregnant or women who are breastfeeding should not participate in 5:2.

- Children and teenagers should not participate in 5:2. They are still developing and growing and therefore need to follow a regular diet without interruption.

- Those who have any other type of medical condition that requires a specific diet, or who have dietary restrictions related to a chronic condition should not participate in 5:2.

Individuals with the above conditions should steer clear of any diet that inflicts extreme diet changes. However, because we don't always do what we should do, I implore you to please consult your physician before embarking on 5:2 or any type of intermittent fasting protocol. Your life and well-being are the most important factors in any given situation.

Counting Calories

Counting calories will make it much easier to lose weight during a diet. However, the thing that makes 5:2, and any intermittent fasting diet so convenient, is that you are not required to count calories every day. You are only really required to count calories on fast days.

That being said, although calorie counting is not required, I absolutely recommend it. Sometimes, people *think* that they are eating within their daily calorie allowance when in reality they may be doubling it, or more! While calorie counting is not mandatory every day of the 5:2, it is a very useful and accurate tool for weight loss, and I recommend it to the fullest!

What is a "Calorie"?

A calorie is actually a unit of heat energy; it is what your body uses to operate. Just as your car needs gasoline to run, your body needs calories. Calories are provided through the food we eat in the form of fat, protein, and carbohydrates.

Factors such as gender, age, height, weight, and activity level determine how many calories our bodies need to function each day.

Logging Calories:

The easiest way to track calories is by monitoring any caloric activity. A great way to do this is by creating a "calorie" section in your 5:2 Diet journal and logging:

1. **The amount of calories entering your body (food/beverages, etc.)**
2. **The amount of calories exiting your body (exercise/activities/sleep)**

Trying to Lose Weight – More calories need to be exiting your body than entering it every day in order for you to be able to *lose* weight.
Trying to Maintain Weight – An equal number of calories need to be entering and exiting your body each day in order for you to be able to *maintain* your current body weight.
Trying to Gain Weight – I know most of us wish we had this problem! More calories need to be entering your body than exiting your body each day in order for you to be able to *gain* weight.
Calories in Food:

Here is the basic breakdown of how calories are divided in a food product:
Fat: 9 Calories Per 1 gram
Protein: 4 Calories Per 1 gram
Carbohydrates: 4 Calories Per 1 gram

So, let's say you are eating a:

Nature Valley Oats 'n Honey Crunchy Granola Bar

Nutrition Facts
Serving Size: 2 bars (42g)
Servings Per Container: 6

Amount Per Serving	2 bars	%DV*	1 bar	%DV*
Calories	186		90	
Calories from Fat	60		30	
Total Fat	6g	9%	3g	5%
Saturated Fat	0.5g	3%	0g	0%
Trans Fat	0g		0g	
Cholesterol	0mg	0%	0mg	0%
Sodium	160mg	7%	80mg	3%
Total Carbohydrate	29g	10%	15g	5%
Dietary Fiber	2g	8%	1g	4%
Sugars	12g		6g	
Protein	4g		2g	
Iron		4%		2%

Not a significant source of vitamin A, vitamin C, and calcium

*Percent Daily Values (DV) are based on a 2,000 calorie diet. Your daily values may be higher or lower depending on your calorie needs.

	Calories	2,000	2,500
Total Fat	Less Than	65g	80g
Sat Fat	Less Than	20g	25g
Cholesterol	Less Than	300mg	300mg
Sodium	Less Than	2,400mg	2,400mg
Total Carbohydrate		300g	375g
Dietary Fiber		25g	30g

When you have the nutrition facts it is easy to determine how many calories you are eating. All of the work is done for you. You know that with nutrition labels, you will already have all that is needed to count calories laid out in front of you, such as serving size, calories, calories, fat, carbs, and protein.

But, what if you only had the serving size, fat grams, carbs, and protein? How would you figure out the calories? To figure it out, we are going to look at the granola bar nutrition facts again – only this time without the calorie information. We are only going to look at the data needed to determine calories, so we are going to get rid of all the other info.

We are going to use the "2 bar" serving size

Nutrition Facts
Serving Size: 2 bars (42g)

Amount Per Serving	2 bars		1 bar	
		%DV*		%DV*
Total Fat	6g	9%	3g	5%
Total Carbohydrate	29g	10%	15g	5%
Protein	4g		2g	

Do you remember how we broke down calories before?
Fat: 9 Calories Per 1 gram
Protein: 4 Calories Per 1 gram
Carbohydrates: 4 Calories Per 1 gram

We know that we are going to eat 2 bars so our:

Serving Size: 2 Bars
We know from the nutritional data that there is **6g Total Fat** per **2 bar serving size.** Above we see that the calorie breakdown for Fat is **9 calories per 1 gram.** So in order to figure out the calories from Total Fat, we are going to **multiply the Total Fat by 9 calories.**

Total Fat: 6g (6 x 9 = 54) **54 Calories**

Now, we are going to figure out the Carbs and Protein in the same way. Look at the Carbs and Protein Data. We know that for Carbs and Protein, the caloric breakdown is the same – **4 calories per 1 gram**:

Total Carbohydrates: 29g (29 x 4 = 116) **116 Calories**
Protein: 4g (4 x 4 = 16) **16 Calories**

Finally, we add the calorie totals from the Total Fat, Carbs, and Protein to come up with the total calories for our serving size:
54 + 116 + 16 = 186 Total Calories for the "2 bar" serving size.

The Do's and Don'ts of Counting Calories

In order to get the most out of counting calories and to ensure that you are counting your calories in a thorough and accurate way, refer to the following Do's and Don'ts of Calorie Counting:

DO remember to count beverage and condiment calories as well. It can be very easy for someone to forget to count beverage and condiment calories. For instance:

- *Someone may count the calories for everything that is in their salad, but they forget to count the salad dressing calories.*
- *Someone may count the calories for their salad as well as the calories for their salad dressing, but they forget to account for the calories of the soft drink that accompanied their salad.*

These miscellaneous calories can be very easy to forget. Let's say your total allowed daily caloric allowance is 1690. At the end of the day, you may be right at 1690 or even under and you think "Woo hoo! That wasn't so bad!" but then you realize that you didn't account for the coffee and syrup at breakfast, the iced tea and ketchup at lunch, the smoothie and whipped cream for snack, and the milk and sour cream you had at dinner. When you add these all to your previous total – you can find that you are 500 or 600 calories OVER your calorie budget!

Beverage and condiment calories are sneaky! They add up quickly and they can blindside you when you think you're right on track with your calories. These calories are just as important as your food calories, so ALWAYS count them when you consume them so that they don't creep up on you at day's end!

Note: This includes little nibbles throughout the day, too. If you grab a handful of cheese crackers, it counts! If you eat a couple bites of macaroni 'n' cheese off your child's plate – it counts! If you eat a few chocolate chips out of the bag – it *also* counts!

Don't rely on memory! This is a biggie. Let's say you are out to lunch with friends and you don't have your calorie journal, notebook, or other way of logging your calories, so you tell yourself "Oh, I will just write them down later this evening – I'll remember!" Well, if you are like most people, you WON'T remember and that whole chunk of calories will not be accounted for, which can easily make it so you go over your daily calorie budget. This jeopardizes your weight loss.

If you don't have your usual calorie log with you, there are other things you can do, such as write the food items/calories on the back of your lunch receipt, or text yourself the calorie total. If you have a home answering machine/voice mail, call and leave a message stating the food items and/or calories that you consumed. Not logging your calories at all is NEVER a good idea. Don't rely on your memory – your weight loss success depends on keeping accurate records!

Do invest in a calorie-counting/logging phone application or electronic database. You will not believe how much easier this will make your life. Phone apps, such as those made for Apple or

Android are the best to use; most of them are free and they come equipped with an extensive food database. If you just ate a banana and type the word "banana" into the application, different options for serving sizes (small, medium, large banana; ½ medium banana-sliced,and so on) as well as the nutrition facts, including calorie info for said serving size, will pop up.

These applications will usually let you track calories being expended through exercise and other activities. There is usually an activity database, like the nutrition database – if you type in the word "cardio" – a list of all types of cardiovascular exercise will pop up (walking, running treadmill, etc). A calorie logging database will save you so much time. One database that is very popular and is available for both Apple and Android is My Fitness Pal – it is a wonderful application with over 10 million users!

Don't attempt to "GUESS" portion sizes. It is very important that your calories are accurate – especially during your Fast-Days. If you guesstimate a portion size, you may be way off track. I know that there are comparisons out there that help you to visualize portions – such as:

- 3-ounces of Chicken or Meat = a deck of cards
- 1½-ounces of cheese = 3 dice
- 1-cup of cooked vegetables = a baseball

You get the idea. While this is okay some of the time – it is NEVER okay for when you are on a diet or trying to lose weight. You need your calorie counts to be precise - therefore, your portions must also be precise. Get a food scale/digital scale – they work amazingly well; use measuring cups and measuring spoons. You can also use pre-portioned food products. However you choose to divide up proper portion sizes, just make sure that you are using an accurate method – NOT YOUR EYES!

Part 3: 5:2 Diet Recipes

Recipes Under 150 Calories

Breakfast Recipes

GARDEN FRESH BREAKFAST TARTS

Delicious little tarts with the ability to keep you full and satisfied until lunchtime. These little tarts are packed full of fluffy, farm-fresh eggs, a variety of veggies, and finely shredded mozzarella.

Prep to finish: 20 - 25 minutes
Difficulty: Easy
Yield: 6 Servings
Serving Size: 2 tarts

Ingredients:
- 1/4 c. milk
- 1 large egg
- 3 large egg whites
- ½ tsp. fresh ground black pepper
- ½ tsp. sea salt
- ¼ c. broccoli, chopped
- ½ clove garlic, minced
- 2 medium mushrooms, chopped
- ½ small whole tomato, diced
- ¼ to ½ c. Italian-style bread crumbs
- ¼ c. mozzarella, finely shredded

Instructions:
1. Begin by prepping 12-cup muffin pan. Use silicon trays if you can. They will do a better job at preventing the eggs from sticking. If using regular pans, grease cups well with cooking spray. Preheat oven to 325 °F.
2. Begin placing the crust by using a teaspoon and scooping a thin, even layer of breadcrumbs into the bottom of each muffin cup. Press the breadcrumbs down to create a muffin base that is ¼-inch thick.
3. Crack the eggs into a medium-sized bowl, add milk and beat well. Set aside. Prepare all of the vegetables and the mozzarella cheese by chopping, dicing, mincing, and shredding each according to the ingredient list. Combine the vegetables together in a separate bowl. Set cheese aside.
4. Pour half of the egg mixture into the bowl of vegetables and mix well. Divide the veggie mixture among each muffin cup by spooning a bit of the mixture over the bread crumb

base. Fill the muffin cups ¾ of the way full. Next, pour a little of the remaining egg mixture into each cup. If you need more, you may crack 1 more egg and 1/16 cup of milk and beat. However, do your best to spread the remaining egg mixture sparingly enough that you are able to fill each cup.

5. Finally, top each muffin cup with one teaspoon of finely-shredded mozzarella cheese. Let the tarts sit out for at least 10 minutes so that the egg mixture has time to seep into the breadcrumbs in order to seal the crust. Transfer muffin pan to the oven and bake at 325 °F for 5 to 7 minutes or until the tarts are golden brown on top and the cheese is melted. Place two tarts on a plate and sprinkle salt and pepper to taste. Enjoy hot.

Nutritional info:
- Calories: 66
- Total Fat: 1.9g
- Total Carbohydrates: 5.2g
- Dietary Fiber: 0.7g
- Sugars: 1. 4g
- Protein: 0g
- Sodium: 6.6mg

BANANA OAT GRANOLA BARS

Crunchy granola bars filled with sliced almonds, chewy raisins and a sweet hint of ripe banana and warm-scented cinnamon. Make a bunch and freeze for on-the-go breakfast and snacks for anytime of the day.

Prep to finish: Prep - 15 minutes; Cook - 45 minutes; Total Time - 1 hour
Difficulty: Easy
Yield: 2 dozen bars
Serving Size: 2 bars

Ingredients:
- 4 large egg whites
- 2 tsp. ground cinnamon
- 1 1/2 medium bananas, overripe
- 1/2 cup packed raisins (optional)
- 1/2 cup sliced almonds
- 2 cups rolled oats

Instructions:
1. Preheat oven to 350 °F.
2. Begin by cracking eggs and separating the egg whites from the yolks. Transfer the egg whites to a medium-sized mixing bowl and discard yolks.
3. Mash banana and mix in with egg whites. Add cinnamon and blend well.
4. Fold in oats, raisins, and almonds. Make sure all ingredients are well blended.
5. Pour granola mixture into a 9" square baking pan. Line pan with parchment paper for easy clean-up.
6. Spread the mixture out across the bottom of the pan and then level the mixture so that the bars are about ¼- to ½-inch thick. Transfer to oven and bake at 350°F for 35 to 40 minutes, or until the bars golden brown.
7. Let bars cool for at least 15 minutes before slicing. Serving size: 2 bars.
8. Note: You can substitute the almonds and raisins for ingredients of choice. Try a variety of nuts and seeds, dried cranberries, organic chocolate chips, etc. Keep in mind that calories and nutrition facts will differ.

Nutritional info:
- Calories: 88
- Total Fat: 1.9g
- Total Carbohydrates: 15.3g
- Dietary Fiber: 2.2g
- Sugars: 3.9g
- Protein: 3.5g
- Sodium: 10mg

CINNAMON PEAR FRENCH CRÊPES

Super-simple french crêpes switched up a bit for a healthful version which is still delectably-tasty. The delicate, thin pancakes are filled with sweet pear and cinnamon. A perfect breakfast for when you have the time to treat yourself! Hint: substitute the pear and cinnamon with a sweeter filling for a succulent dessert. Bon Appetit!

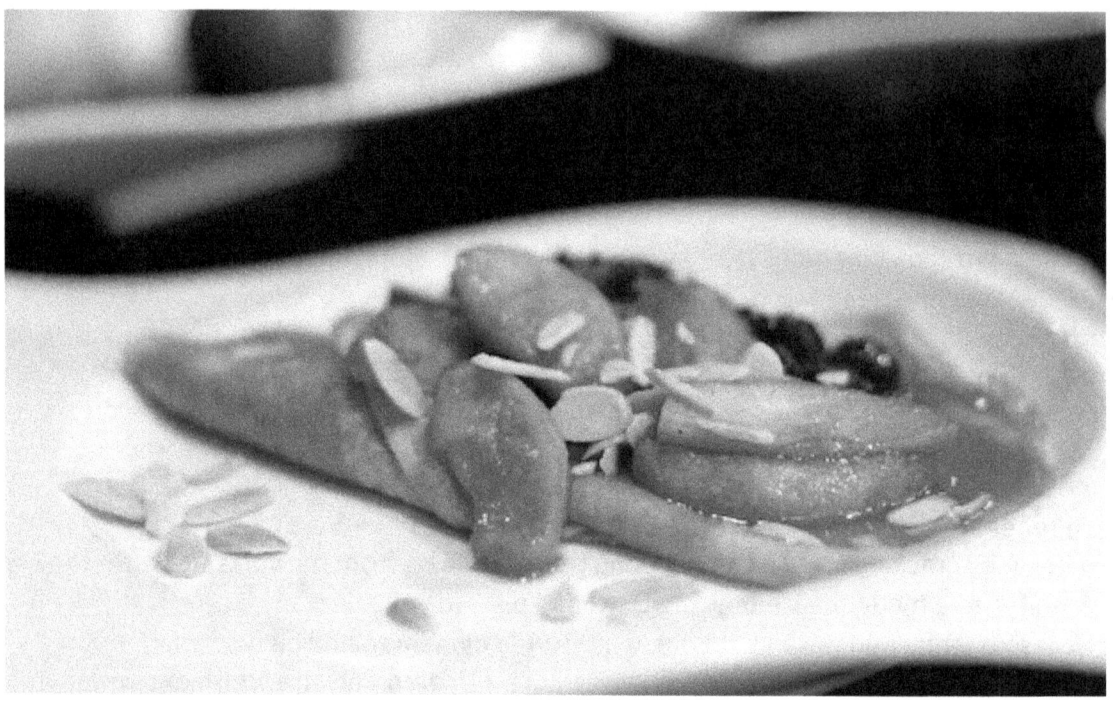

Prep to finish: Prep - 5 minutes; Cook - 30 minutes; Total Time - 35 minutes
Difficulty: Medium
Yield: 2 servings
Serving Size: 2 crêpes

Ingredients:
Batter
- 1/2 c. whole wheat flour
- 2/3 c. nonfat milk
- 2 Eggs
- 1 tsp. sugar
- ¼ tsp. baking powder
- 2 tbsp. butter or margarine (melted and cooled)
- Pinch of Salt
- ¼ tsp. vanilla bean scrapings (optional)
- Extra virgin olive oil (can use olive oil spray, if preferred) for pan

Filling
- ¾ c. water
- ¾ tsp. plus 1 tsp. cinnamon
- ¼ tbsp. butter or margarine
- 2 pears, peeled and cut into cubes or slices

Instructions:
1. To begin, melt butter or margarine and set aside to let cool.
2. Sift whole wheat flour into a medium-sized mixing bowl. Mix in salt. Add in sugar and baking soda. Blend well.
3. Form a well in the center of the bowl. Add eggs to the center of the well and stir ingredients together. Slowly pour in milk, stirring constantly until small bubbles appear on surface of the batter. Finally, stir in melted butter or margarine. Note: you want the batter to be thin. If it seems thicker – like a cream consistency – add a little water or milk.
4. Prepare the filling: place the water and pears in a pan over medium-high heat. When most of the liquid has vanished and the pears are cooked, stir in ¼ tbsp. butter or margarine.
5. Place an 8-inch skillet, coated or sprayed with olive oil, over high-heat. Note: Make sure that pan is completely coated! Place 2 to 3 tbsp. of batter onto skillet and quickly move skillet around in order for the batter to spread evenly. You want the cover the enter bottom of the skillet with a thin layer of batter.
6. Let cook for 1 minute or until golden brown, then flip the crêpe with spatula and continue cooking for 30 more seconds or until golden brown. Place 2 crêpes on a plate, top one-half of each crêpe with the pear filling. Top the pear filling by dusting it with a little cinnamon. Fold the bare half over the filled half. Serve immediately!

Nutritional info:
- Calories: 119
- Total Fat: 5 g
- Total Carbohydrates: 18g
- Dietary Fiber: 3g
- Sugars: 7g
- Protein: 4g
- Sodium: 70mg

VEGETARIAN BREAKFAST FRITTATA

Fluffy eggs meet only the freshest garden veggies in this breakfast dish that is as filling as it is delicious. Quick and simple to make, this vitamin-rich, low-calorie, low-carb dish is packed with protein to keep you going strong until your next meal. Finally, you can have a hot restaurant-style breakfast in just a matter of minutes, even on those days you find yourself rushing out the door! Note: For a non-vegetarian version, use the chicken sausage as noted in the ingredients.

Prep to finish: Prep time - 5 minutes; Cook time - 6 to 8 minutes; Total time – 11 to 13 minutes
Difficulty: Easy
Yield: 2 servings
Serving Size: 2 slices

Ingredients:
- 1 medium egg (opt.)
- 3 large egg whites (if not using whole egg, use 4 large egg whites)
- ½ clove garlic, minced
- 1 sprig fresh cilantro
- ¼ c. broccoli, chopped
- 2 medium mushrooms, chopped
- ½ small whole tomato, diced
- 1 tbsp. red onion, chopped fine
- ¼ to ½ c. Italian-style bread crumbs
- ¼ c. mozzarella, finely shredded
- ½ tsp. fresh ground black pepper
- ½ tsp. sea salt
- Olive oil non-stick cooking spray

For a non-vegetarian version:
- 2/3 c. chicken sausage, crumbled

Instructions:
1. Preheat oven to 350 °F.
2. Spray a black cast-iron skillet with non-stick cooking spray. Make sure the skillet is well coated. Place skillet over low-heat.
3. While the skillet is heating up, prepare vegetables as instructed above. Place the onions and garlic in the skillet and sauté for a moment until the garlic is fragrant and the onions, translucent. Stir in broccoli, tomatoes, and (if using) the crumbled sausage. Sauté for about 1 minute, stirring constantly. Remove skillet from heat.
4. In a small bowl, combine the egg whites, whole egg, salt, and pepper and beat well. Pour egg mixture over vegetables in skillet. Stir to make sure the vegetables are well blended throughout the egg mixture. Sprinkle the finely shredded mozzarella and torn cilantro over the surface of the frittata.

5. Transfer to oven and let cook at 350 for 6 – 8 minutes or until the eggs are set and cheese is melted. Remove from oven and let sit for one minute. Slice the frittata in half and then slice it in half again, so that there are 4 slices. Transfer 2 slices to a serving dish and enjoy!

Nutritional info:
- Calories: 60
- Total Fat: 0.8g
- Total Carbohydrates: 4.5g
- Dietary Fiber: 1.2g
- Sugars: 1.6g
- Protein: 8.9g
- Sodium: 263mg

TANGY MANGO MUFFINS

A super low-calorie, extra-delicious muffin that will spoil your palate and tickle your taste buds. The sweet taste of mango and banana packed into these light and fluffy muffins make a combination that is delectably dangerous – yet will keep you on task with your weight loss efforts. These muffins are good for those on-the-go with little time to spare! Try making a few dozen and freezing them – just pop them in the microwave when you want one or let them sit out to thaw out!

Prep to finish: 50 minutes
Difficulty: Medium
Yield: 1 dozen muffins
Serving Size: 1 muffin

Ingredients:
- 1 1/4 c. whole wheat flour
- 1/4 c. all-purpose flour
- 1/8 tsp. baking powder
- 3/4 tsp. baking soda
- 2 tsp. cinnamon
- 1/2 c. sugar
- 1/2 tsp. salt
- 3 large egg whites
- 1/4 c. apple sauce
- ½ tbsp. lime juice
- 1/8 c. orange juice, no-pulp
- 1 tsp. vanilla
- 1 medium banana, sliced or mashed
- 1 c. fresh mango, sliced
- 1/2 c. walnuts, finely chopped

Tools:
- 12 cup muffin pan
- 12 paper muffin liners or olive oil cooking spray

Instructions:
1. Preheat oven to 350 °F.
2. In a large mixing bowl, combine both flours, baking powder, baking soda, cinnamon, sugar, and salt.
3. In a separate medium-sized mixing bowl, combine the egg whites, apple sauce, lime juice, orange juice, and vanilla. Mix well. Add the egg mixture to the dry ingredients and stir, blending thoroughly.
4. Finally, stir in the banana, mango, and nuts.

5. Fill a 12-cup muffin pan with paper muffin liners. NOTE: If you are not using paper liners, spray the cups with olive oil cooking spray, until each cup is well coated.
6. Fill the muffin cups with muffin batter until each cup is two-thirds of the way full. Transfer pan to oven and bake at 350 °F for 20-25 minutes, or until a toothpick inserted into the center of a muffin comes out clean.
7. Let muffins sit for 5 minutes before transferring to wire racks.
8. Muffins can be enjoyed hot or cold.

Nutritional info:
- Calories: 98
- Total Fat: 0.3g
- Total Carbohydrates: 21.9g
- Dietary Fiber: 1.8g
- Sugars: 9.2g
- Protein: 2.8g
- Sodium: 248mg

CINNAMON PUMPKIN PANCAKES

For a special treat, whip up some of these healthfully scrumptious cinnamon pumpkin pancakes. These light and fluffy cakes are packed full of just the right amount of spices to make this a filling and delicious breakfast for the whole family. These are perfect for a crisp Fall morning or for any time of the year!

Prep to finish: 15 minutes
Difficulty: Easy
Yield: 4 servings
Serving Size: 3 pancakes (4-inch diameter)

Ingredients:
- 1 c. nonfat milk (or soy milk, if preferred)
- 1 large egg
- 1/2 tsp. cinnamon
- 1/2 tsp. ginger
- 1/4 tsp. nutmeg
- 1/4 tsp. salt
- 1 tbsp. canola oil
- 1/3 c. pumpkin
- 1 1/2 tsp. baking powder
- 1/2 c. brown sugar
- 1 c. flour

Instructions:
1. Preheat skillet over medium heat.
2. In a medium-sized mixing bowl, mix together all the dry ingredients. Blend thoroughly.
3. In a second, smaller mixing bowl, combine together all the wet ingredients. Blend thoroughly.
4. Add the wet ingredients to the dry ingredients and stir until all ingredients are well blended.
5. Drop ¼ cup of batter at a time onto the preheated skillet to make pancakes that are approximately 4 inches in diameter.
6. Cook pancakes for approximately 1½- 2 minutes or until golden brown. Flip the pancakes over using spatula and continue cooking for approximately 1½-2 minutes on other side, or until golden brown.
7. Transfer three pancakes to a serving plate.
8. TOPPINGS: Optional - top pancakes with your choice of fresh fruit, syrup, peanut butter, or other topping. Be sure to include the additional calories for any toppings you may use!!!

Nutritional info:
- Calories: 98
- Total Fat: 2.4g
- Total Carbohydrates: 16.7g
- Dietary Fiber: 0.8g
- Sugars: 6.2g
- Protein: 2.6g
- Sodium: 154mg

Lunch Recipes

BABY SPINACH AND SHRIMP SALAD

This is a light, yet filling salad that is perfect for an early or late lunch. Healthy and delicious, this salad provides a well-balanced meal to keep you going strong, especially during Fast-Days. Try grilling the shrimp for a crispier texture!

Prep to finish: 5 minutes
Difficulty: Easy
Yield: 1serving
Serving Size: 1 salad

Ingredients:
- 1 tsp. garlic powder
- 1 tbsp. balsamic dressing, low fat
- 1 cup spinach
- 6 small shrimp, cooked (boiled or grilled)

Instructions:
1. If spinach is raw, wash well. Grill or boil shrimp until cooked through.
2. Place raw baby spinach in a small bowl. Sprinkle the spinach with garlic and balsamic dressing. Toss to coat.
3. Arrange baby spinach leaves on a salad dish. Top with grilled or boiled shrimp. Enjoy!

Nutritional info:
- Calories: 59
- Total Fat: 1.6g
- Total Carbohydrates: 4.1g
- Dietary Fiber: 1g
- Sugars: 1.5g
- Protein: 7.5g
- Sodium: 274mg

GREEK YOGURT TOPPED CHICKPEA VEGGIE BURGERS

These protein-packed veggie burgers will leave you feeling satisfied and ready to take on the rest of the day. The Greek yogurt makes for a delicious spin on an already great veggie burger - your hunt for the perfect veggie burger is over!

Prep to finish: Prep time - 30 minutes; Total time - 50 minutes
Difficulty: Medium
Yield: 4 servings (8 burgers)
Serving Size: 2 burgers

Ingredients:
Burgers
- 2 (15-ounce) cans chickpeas, drained and rinsed
- 2 tsp. garam masala
- 2 tbsp. extra virgin olive oil
- 2 egg whites
- 1/2 c. toasted bread crumbs
- 1/2 c. plain Greek yogurt
- 4 scallions, minced
- 3 tbsp. cilantro, minced
- Sea salt, to taste
- 4 leaves of Bibb lettuce

Yogurt Sauce
- 1 c. plain Greek yogurt
- 1/2 cucumber, shredded
- 2 tbsp. scallions, chopped very fine
- 1 tbsp. fresh cilantro, chopped very fine
- Sea salt

Instructions:
1. To begin, prepare the yogurt sauce. Peel the cucumber and scoop out any seeds using a spoon. Using the larger holes of a grater, begin shredding the cucumber into a colander. Sprinkle a 1/8 tsp. sea salt on the shredded cucumber, toss to coat, and set cucumber aside for 10 to 15 minutes. Be sure to place paper towels or a dish towel under the colander, as the vegetable will lose moisture while it sits.
2. While waiting for your cucumber to set, take a medium-sized mixing bowl and add 1 c. Greek yogurt, scallions, and 1 tbsp. of cilantro – remember to make sure that scallions and cilantro are very finely chopped. Add shredded cucumber to the bowl and stir until the yogurt sauce is smooth and thick. Place your sauce in the refrigerator until it is needed.
3. Prepare burgers. First, place breadcrumbs in a pan and place over medium heat. Toast for 5 minutes until the breadcrumbs are golden brown. Make sure to not burn them – remove from heat. Meanwhile, in a small bowl, combine egg whites, garam masala, olive

oil, and a pinch of sea salt. Whisk the ingredients together well. The mixture may look a bit odd, but it will smell great!

4. In a separate large mixing bowl, add your drained and rinsed chickpeas and mash them up really well. They can be as chunky or smooth as you like. Add your egg mixture and toasted breadcrumbs to the mashed chickpeas. Blend thoroughly. Next, add in your 1 c. Greek yogurt, scallions, and cilantro. Blend thoroughly.

5. Place a skillet or frying pan over medium-high to high heat. Add 2 tbsp. olive oil to the skillet/pan or coat with cooking spray. While the skillet is heating up, divide your burger mixture into 8 equal parts and form patties that are about ¾" thick. Place patties in the pan or on the skillet and cook approximately 3 to 5 minutes per side, or until the patties are cooked through and are golden brown. Arrange 2 Bibb lettuce leaves on a serving dish. Place two burger patties on the lettuce leaves. Take your yogurt sauce out of the fridge and top each patty with 1½ to 2 tbsp. of the yogurt sauce. Eat immediately and enjoy!

Nutritional info:
- Calories: 96
- Total Fat: 2.4g
- Total Carbohydrates: 13.6g
- Dietary Fiber: 5.3g
- Sugars: 2.1g
- Protein: 5.8g
- Sodium: mg

Spinach Portobello Pizza Caps

The deliciously fun and tasty little bite-size pizzas provide a fully-packed, nutritional powerhouse of a meal. Who would have thought that so much nutritional value could be wrapped up in such tiny little packages? Don't let their size fool you! They may be small, but they will keep you feeling full and satisfied as if you had just enjoyed a 5-course meal – these little guys are a restricted calorie faster's dream come true!

Prep to finish: Prep time - 10 minutes; Cook time – 10 to 12 minutes; Total time – 20 to 22 minutes
Difficulty: Easy
Yield: 2 servings (4 caps)
Serving Size: 2 caps

Ingredients:
- 4 Portobello mushroom caps; washed well, dried, and stems removed
- 1/3 c. tomato sauce
- 1/2 c. baby spinach leaves, torn
- 2/3 tbsp. fresh garlic, minced
- 2 2/3 tbsp. black olives, sliced
- 2 2/3 tbsp. green bell pepper, sliced (or can be cut into chunks or diced)
- 2 2/3 tbsp. red onion, chopped
- A few cherry tomatoes, sliced (use preferred amount for each pizza)
- 1/2 c. mozzarella cheese, finely shredded (will use 2 tbsp. per pizza)
- 15 spinach leaves
- Fresh or dried basil, to garnish (opt.)
- 1/4 tbsp. dried Italian seasonings

Instructions:
1. Preheat oven to 375°F. Line a baking sheet with parchment paper.
2. Place each mushroom, cap side up, on the baking sheet and place in oven to bake for 5 minutes.
3. While the mushrooms are baking, place the tomato sauce in a small, shallow bowl. Add dried Italian seasonings and blend well. Prepare other ingredients as directed.
4. Remove mushroom caps from oven and spoon or brush the tomato sauce over the center of each cap. Next, layer each cap with 2 tbsp. of finely shredded mozzarella, followed by a few baby spinach leaves, cherry tomatoes, olives, green bell pepper, chopped red onion, and garlic.
5. Place caps in oven and bake 12 to 15 minutes or until cheese is melted and edges are golden. Garnish each pizza cap with fresh or dried basil (optional) and transfer two caps to a serving dish. Enjoy while hot!

Nutritional info:
- Calories: 98
- Total Fat: 3.7g
- Total Carbohydrates: 8.3g
- Dietary Fiber: 3g
- Sugars: 2.3g
- Protein: 7.6g
- Sodium: 238mg

RADICCHIO, ORANGE, AND ARUGULA SALAD

This tangy and citrusy salad is loaded with Vitamin C and antioxidants. It is a great salad for fast days, as it provides a nutritious punch for your body, despite the reduction in calorie intake. The arugula accompanies the citrusy sweetness perfectly and the crunchy toasted walnuts really bring this taste home – this is a salad you will find yourself making often!

Prep to finish: 5 minutes
Difficulty: Easy
Yield: 1 serving
Serving Size: 1 salad

Ingredients:
- 1 medium-size seedless orange; peeled and sectioned, then sliced and cut into chunks
- 1 tbsp. pulp-free orange juice
- 1 tbsp. extra virgin olive oil
- ½ tbsp. white wine vinegar
- 1 tsp. walnut oil
- ¼ tsp. orange peel, grated
- 1/2 medium-size head radicchio, torn into bite-size pieces
- 1/2 bunch arugula, washed and ends trimmed
- 1/8 c. walnuts, toasted and chopped

Instructions:
6. To begin, place walnuts in a pan over medium-high heat and toast walnuts.
7. Using a sharp knife - peel orange and cut away the white pith. Cut oranges crosswise into 1/4-inch thick slices and then cut each slice in half. Set aside.
8. In a medium-sized mixing bowl, whisk together orange juice, olive oil, vinegar, walnut oil and grated orange peel. Season with salt and pepper.
9. In a separate large bowl, combine radicchio, arugula and orange slices in large bowl. Add vinegar; toss to coat greens.
10. Place in salad bowl and sprinkle with 1/8 c. chopped toasted walnuts.

Nutritional info:
- Calories: 84
- Total Fat: 5.6g
- Total Carbohydrates: 6.7g
- Dietary Fiber: 2.8g
- Sugars: 4.9g
- Protein: 3.5g
- Sodium: 308mg

SPINACH AND MUSHROOM-STUFFED MANICOTTI

Fresh spinach and mushrooms combined with ricotta and mozzarella cheeses and stuffed into tender manicotti pasta with a hint of tomato sauce makes this one lunch you won't forget anytime soon – plus it's a pasta dish under 100 calories – need we say more?!

Prep to finish: Prep time – 5 minutes; Cook time – 50 minutes
Difficulty: Medium
Yield: 2 servings
Serving Size: 2 stuffed manicotti shells

Ingredients:
- ¼ c. low fat ricotta cheese
- ½ c. mozzarella cheese, shredded
- 1/8 c. parmesan cheese, shredded or grated
- (4) manicotti pasta shells
- ½ to ¾ c. tomato sauce or preferred sauce
- ¼ to ½ c. fresh or frozen spinach, chopped fine
- 1/8 c. button mushrooms, washed and chopped or sliced
- ½ tbsp. garlic powder
- ½ tsp. ground oregano
- 1/16 tsp. crushed red pepper (opt.)
- Pinch salt, to taste
- Pinch fresh ground black pepper, to taste
- 1 ½ cups spaghetti sauce
- 2 cups spinach

Instructions:
1. Preheat oven to 350°F.
2. Place a large saucepan, filled 2/3 of the way full with water, over high heat and bring water to a boil. Add a pinch of salt to the water to help prevent the pasta from sticking.
3. When water reaches a rolling boil, add manicotti shells and boil for about 6 minutes or until al dente.
4. While the pasta is boiling, in a medium-sized mixing bowl, combine the ricotta cheese, spinach, mushrooms, and spices. Blend well.
5. Remove pasta from heat, drain carefully, and quickly rinse with cool water. Once the pasta is cool enough for you to touch, lay the shells on the counter on a piece of parchment paper, in order to prevent them from sticking to one another or being crushed in the pan.
6. Fill each shell. Cup the manicotti shell in one hand. With your finger, block one end of the shell. Using a fork or piping bag, stuff each shell with the spinach mixture. Continue stuffing each shell one at a time until all shells have been stuffed.

7. Place the stuffed manicotti shells in a baking dish, coated with olive oil cooking spray. Cover each shell with a little tomato sauce or preferred sauce. Add 1/8 to ¼ c. of water (just enough for the bottom of the baking pan to be covered) to the baking dish. Cover baking dish with aluminum foil and bake at 350°F for 25 minutes. Take out of the oven and remove foil.
8. Sprinkle the stuffed manicotti shells with the shredded mozzarella and parmesan cheeses and return to oven. Continue cooking for approximately 20 more minutes or until the remaining moisture has almost disappeared, the cheeses are melted, and the edges are golden brown.
9. Transfer 2 stuffed manicotti shells to serving dish and enjoy!

Nutritional info:
- Calories: 97
- Total Fat: 3g
- Total Carbohydrates: 12.3g
- Dietary Fiber: 2.3g
- Sugars: 4.8g
- Protein: 5.2g
- Sodium: 149mg

Avocado and Egg White Salad

Boiled egg whites, crisp green apple, and just enough chopped avocado for the sweetness – filling, but not enough to break your calorie budget - makes this a salad worth celebrating! Quick to prepare and a joy to eat – you won't believe something that tastes this good can be so good for you!

Prep to finish: 5 minutes
Difficulty: Easy
Yield: 1serving
Serving Size: 1 salad

Ingredients:

- 2 large egg whites, boiled and chopped
- 2 tbsp. plain Greek yogurt
- 1/2 medium granny smith apple, chopped
- 1/4 avocado, chopped
- 1½ tsp. lemon juice
- 1/2 cup romaine lettuce, or preferred lettuce, chopped
- 3/4 tsp. parsley, minced

Instructions:

1. In a small bowl, combine egg whites, yogurt, apple, avocado, and lemon juice and toss gently as to coat the ingredients well with yogurt and lemon juice.
2. Arrange chopped lettuce on a salad plate and top lettuce with yogurt mixture. Serve immediately.

Nutritional info:
- Calories: 99
- Total Fat: 2.2g
- Total Carbohydrates: 10.2g
- Dietary Fiber: 3.9g
- Sugars: 4.5g
- Protein: 4.7g
- Sodium: 137mg

Snack Recipes

Cinnamon-Spiced Apple Chips

This is a wonderful, healthful snack for anytime of the day. These apples chips are so easy to make, they practically make themselves! Sure, they may take more time from start to finish, but they are SO worth the wait. Try making a large batch and storing them in a freezer bag for a quick, readily-available snack.

Prep to finish: Prep time: 10 minutes; Cook time – 2 hours; Total time – 2 hours 10 minutes
Difficulty: Easy
Yield: 12 servings
Serving Size: 1½ c. apple chips

Ingredients:
- 6 to 8 medium apples
- ½ c. lemon juice
- 1 1/3 tbsp. ground cinnamon

Instructions:
1. Preheat oven to 250°F.
2. Prepare the apples by cutting them into very thin slices, about 1/16" thick. Discard both ends of each apple.
3. Wash apple slices and pat dry.
4. Place apple slices in a sealable freezer bag. Pour the lemon juice and cinnamon into the freezer bag over the apple slices.
5. Seal the bag and shake vigorously as to coat the apple slices in the juice and cinnamon.
6. Transfer coated apple slices on to foil-lined cookie sheet(s). Place in oven and bake at 250°F for 2 hours. Be sure to turn apple slices every 30 minutes!
7. Remove from oven and let cool. Serving size is 1 ½ c. apple chips. Store remaining apple chips in an airtight container for up to 30 days.

Nutritional info:
- Calories: 50
- Total Fat: 0.1g
- Total Carbohydrates: 13.5g
- Dietary Fiber: 2.2g
- Sugars: 9.8g
- Protein: 0.3g
- Sodium: 1mg

STRING CHEESE ROLL-UPS

Here is a protein-packed snack perfect for a midday pick-me-up. Try using your favorite cheeses and meats to change the recipe up a bit. The possibilities are endless!

Prep to finish: 3 minutes
Difficulty: Easy
Yield: 2 servings
Serving Size: 1 roll-up

Ingredients:

- 2 sticks part-skim mozzarella string cheese
- 2 thin slices deli turkey breast
- 5 olives (of choice)
- 1/4 c. grapes (of choice)***
- 2 tbsp. balsamic vinegar

*** Can substitute roasted bell peppers for olives and grapes, if desired

Instructions:

1. Wrap one slice of turkey breast around one stick of mozzarella string cheese and place in a snack dish.
2. Arrange three olives and some grapes around the wrapped cheese.
3. Drizzle 1 tbsp. of balsamic vinegar over the snack. Repeat process for second serving. Serve immediately.

Nutritional info:
- Calories: 135
- Total Fat: 6g
- Total Carbohydrates: 8g
- Dietary Fiber: 0g
- Sugars: 6g
- Protein: 12g
- Sodium: 500mg

GREEK YOGURT WITH CINNAMON MAPLE CRUNCH TOPPING

If you love yogurt parfaits, wait until you take your first bite of this yogurt and topping combo. You will buckle at the knees when you realize that the miraculous mixture you are falling hard for is under 90 calories!

Prep to finish: 5 minutes
Difficulty: Easy
Yield: 2 servings
Serving Size: ½ cup. Greek yogurt and ¼ c. topping

Ingredients:
- 1 c. Greek yogurt, plain or vanilla flavored
- ½ c. almonds
- ½ c. walnuts
- 1 c. shredded coconut, unsweetened
- 1 tbsp. coconut oil
- 1 tsp. cinnamon
- 1 tbsp. maple syrup
- pinch of sea salt, to taste

Instructions:
1. Melt the coconut oil in a pan over medium heat. Add the almonds and walnuts and toss for 1 minute.
2. Add the cinnamon, maple syrup, shredded coconut, and a pinch of sea salt. Blend thoroughly.
3. Sauté ingredients for 2 to 4 minutes or until coconut flakes are slightly browned. Let cool.
4. Scoop 1/2 c. of Greek yogurt into each parfait dish. Top the yogurt with ¼ c. of the topping. Enjoy!

Nutritional info:
- Calories: 89
- Total Fat: 2.3g
- Total Carbohydrates: 13.4g
- Dietary Fiber: 3.6g
- Sugars: 4.9g
- Protein: 4.2g
- Sodium: 320mg

CRISPY KALE CHIPS

Kale chips are becoming very popular — maybe it's the crunch and texture that people love. Maybe it's the fact that they taste great but are still good for you. Maybe it's because they are a mess-free snack for the entire family. Whatever makes kale chips so great — isn't time you find out what the hype's all about for yourself? Here is a great, fail-proof recipe to get you hooked on the kale chip-craze!

Prep to finish: 25 to 30 minutes
Difficulty: Easy
Yield: 4 servings
Serving Size: 1½ c. kale chips

Ingredients:
- 2 tbsp. apple cider vinegar
- 1 tsp. sea salt
- 1 tbsp. extra virgin olive oil
- 6 c. fresh kale, chopped

Instructions:
1. Preheat oven to 350°F.
2. Wash kale, pat dry, and then chop.
3. Place kale in a sealable freezer bag. Add olive oil, seal bag, and toss until kale is evenly coated in oil.
4. Open bag and pour in vinegar. Seal bag and toss again to coat kale.
5. Place kale on sturdy baking sheet and place in preheated oven for 10 minutes. Remove from oven and toss gently to move kale around.
6. Place kale back in oven and bake for an addition 8 to 12 minutes or until the desired crispiness is reached. NOTE: If kale is still soft, but browning too quickly, reduce heat to 325°F and keep a watchful eye.
7. Remove kale chips from oven and sprinkle with sea salt, to taste. Serve hot or wait until cool. Store remaining kale chips in airtight container.

Nutritional info:
- Calories: 80
- Total Fat: 4g
- Total Carbohydrates: 10g
- Dietary Fiber: 2g
- Sugars: 0g
- Protein: 3.3g
- Sodium: 486mg

SALT AND PEPPER POPCORN

This popcorn is so much better than the buttery-mess you see in movie theaters! Next time you are watching a movie, take in some of this delicious popcorn as well. One thing is guaranteed – you will be more into the popcorn than the movie!

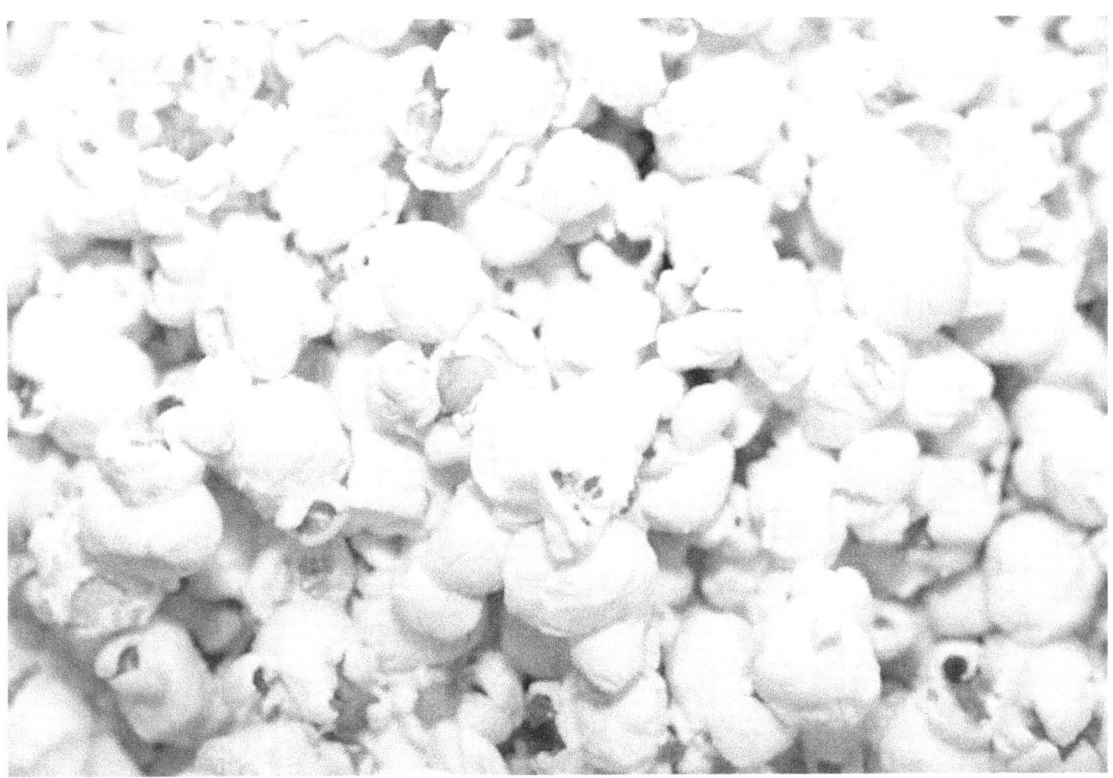

Prep to finish: 5 minutes
Difficulty: Easy
Yield: 1 serving
Serving Size: whole bag

Ingredients:
- ¼ c. organic popcorn kernels
- ½ tsp. pink Himalayan sea salt
- ¼ tsp. fresh ground black pepper
- 2 tsp. extra virgin olive oil

Instructions:
1. Pour popcorn kernels into a brown paper lunch bag. Fold the top of the bag 2 to 3 times to ensure that it will stay closed.
2. Place bag in the microwave and heat for 3 to 3½ minutes on 80% power. Note: microwaves vary, so pay close attention and stop the microwave when there is 1-2

seconds of silence between pops. Popcorn can easily burn – never use the "popcorn" setting on your microwave and walk away.

3. Remove from microwave and open bag. Pour the olive oil, sea salt, and pepper into bag and shake to coat the popcorn well.
4. Pour popcorn into a bowl or enjoy straight out of the bag!

Nutritional info:
- Calories: 100
- Total Fat: 5.8g
- Total Carbohydrates: 13g
- Dietary Fiber: 2.5g
- Sugars: 0g
- Protein: 2g
- Sodium: 253mg

TOMATO-FIG BRUSCHETTA

You have probably tried the classic tomato and basil bruschetta – but just wait until you sink your teeth into this new spin on a beloved classic. You will be rejoicing over the fig and wondering why it took so long to be introduced to your now thankful palate. Filled with protein and slow-digesting ingredients – this snack will help keep you going between meals on fast days.

Prep to finish: 20 minutes
Difficulty: Easy
Yield: 6 servings
Serving Size: 4 slices

Ingredients:
- 12 thin slices of whole-wheat French bread
- 1 clove garlic, for rubbing
- 2 to 3 tomatoes, sliced thin
- 3 figs, each cut into 8 small wedges
- 8 to 10 fresh basil leaves, chiffanade
- Sea salt and fresh ground black pepper, to taste
- 1-2 tsp. balsamic vinegar

Instructions:
1. Preheat oven to 400°F.
2. Slice bread into 12 thin slices and place on a cookie sheet. Bake bread in preheated oven for 5 to 8 minutes or until bread is lightly toasted.
3. Remove bread from oven and immediately rub garlic clove on each slice, to give it the aroma and fresh taste of garlic.
4. Cut each slice of bread in half. You should now have 24 pieces. Place a tomato slice and one fig wedge onto each piece of bread.
5. Sprinkle each piece of bread with salt and pepper, to taste.
6. Drizzle vinegar over each slice and top off with basil.
7. Serve immediately. Serving size: 4 pieces of bruschetta.

Nutritional info:
- Calories: 100
- Total Fat: 1.4g
- Total Carbohydrates: 18.2g
- Dietary Fiber: 3.1g
- Sugars: 2.7g
- Protein: 4.1g
- Sodium: 298mg

WATERMELON-LIME SALSA

A sweet, crunchy, and refreshing snack that is as good by itself or with chips as it is alongside grilled chicken or fish. This is versatile snack that can be whipped up within a matter of minutes, but the taste will have people believing that you slaved away for hours on this sweet and savory salsa mixture. As a plus, watermelon contains arginine, a compound that helps with weight loss!

Prep to finish: 20 minutes
Difficulty: Easy
Yield: 2 servings
Serving Size: ½ c. salsa

Ingredients:
- 1 to 1½ c. watermelon, finely diced
- ½ jalapeno pepper, seeded and minced
- 1 1/3 tbsp. fresh cilantro, chopped
- 1 tbsp. lime juice
- 1 tbsp. red onion, minced
- Sea salt, to taste
- 20 tortilla chips

Instructions:
1. In a medium-sized mixing bowl, combine watermelon, minced jalapeno, cilantro, lime juice, and red onion. Stir until well blended.
2. Sprinkle with sea salt, to taste.
3. Place 1/2 c. salsa and enjoy. Try alongside tortilla or kale chips.
4. Any remaining salsa can be covered and stored in the refrigerator for up to 24-hours.

Nutritional info
- Calories: 32
- Total Fat: 0g
- Total Carbohydrates: 7g
- Dietary Fiber: 1g
- Sugar: 4.2g
- Protein: 1g
- Sodium: 75mg

ORANGE-BERRY FROZEN YOGURT

When you are craving a frozen treat, whip up some of this easy to make frozen yogurt, which is blissfully tasty from first to last bite. Strawberries, orange juice, and creamy yogurt are the main players in this satisfying Vitamin C-packed treat!

Prep to finish: Prep time: 15 minutes; Total time – 2 hours 45 minutes
Difficulty: Easy
Yield: 2 servings
Serving Size: ½ c. frozen yogurt

Ingredients:
- 1 1/3 c. strawberries, hulled
- 1 3/4 tbsp. sugar (may use Truvia or other sugar substitute, if preferred)
- 2 tsp. orange juice, no pulp
- ½ c. Greek yogurt, plain

Instructions:
1. Begin by hulling strawberries – to do so, wash strawberries and then take a small, sharp knife and cut around the leafy top of the strawberry in a circular motion. Remove the stem and leaves and discard.
2. Place the hulled strawberries in a food processor and pulse until smooth, scraping down the sides with a spoon or spatula, as needed.
3. Add sugar and orange juice. Process for a few more seconds to blend the ingredients together.
4. Add yogurt and pulse all ingredients together for few more seconds until well blended.
5. Place yogurt mixture in a bowl, cover with plastic wrap and refrigerate for at least an hour, preferably 2 hours.
6. Transfer mixture to an ice cream maker and process. Serve immediately.

Nutritional info:
- Calories: 84
- Total Fat: 0g
- Total Carbohydrates: 20g
- Dietary Fiber: 2g
- Sugars: 3.8g
- Protein: 1g
- Sodium: 12mg

CHEERIOS TRAIL MIX

There are so many endless possibilities when it comes to snacking on trail mix. Try this yummy mixture of Cheerios, pumpkin seeds, raisins, and chocolate chips for a fun snack the whole family will love. Just prepare to make large batches because this enjoyable blend of nutritional goodness will fly off the counter!

Prep to finish: 10 minutes
Difficulty: Easy
Yield: 12 servings
Serving Size: 1/2 c.

Ingredients:
- ¾ c. Cheerios cereal
- ¾ c. pumpkin seeds (or sunflower seeds, if preferred)
- ½ c. raisins
- ½ c. semisweet min chocolate chips

Instructions:
1. In a sealable freezer bag, combine Cheerios, pumpkin seeds, raisins, and mini chocolate chips.
2. Seal bag and shake to blend.
3. Serving size: ½ c. trail mix. Remaining trail mix can be stored in airtight container for up to one month.

Nutritional info:
- Calories: 98
- Total Fat: 3g
- Total Carbohydrates: 15.6g
- Dietary Fiber: 2g
- Sugars: 3.9g
- Protein: 2g
- Sodium: 78mg

COCOA COCONUT BANANAS

Toasted flaked coconut, sweet cocoa, and vitamin-rich bananas wrapped up in an 80-calorie snack is absolutely a cause for celebration! Loaded with Vitamin B6, Vitamin C, Potassium and other key nutrients and minerals – you will be rewarding your body and your taste buds simultaneously!

Prep to finish: 10 minutes
Difficulty: Easy
Yield: 2 servings
Serving Size: 4 banana pieces

Ingredients:
- 1 to 2 medium bananas, peeled
- 2 tsp. cocoa powder
- 2 tbsp. unsweetened coconut, toasted

Instructions:
1. Preheat oven to 350°F.
2. Place coconut on baking sheet. Place coconut in oven and toast about 20 minutes or until coconut flakes are a golden brown and lightly toasted.
3. While the coconut is in the oven, prepare the banana. To do so, peel and cut at a bias. This means that instead of cutting straight across, cut the banana at a 45-degree angle. Try to cut pieces that are approximately 1-inch thick. Cut 1 to 2 bananas, until you are left with (8) angled, 1-1½" thick slices.
4. Place the cocoa and toasted coconut into two separate small, shallow bowls. Take each banana piece and first roll it in the cocoa and then dip one side of the banana into the coconut. Lay on a serving dish, toasted coconut side-up. Repeat process until all 8 banana slices have been rolled and dipped.
5. Serve immediately. Serving size: 4 pieces.

Nutritional info:
- Calories: 80
- Total Fat: 1g
- Total Carbohydrates: 19g
- Dietary Fiber: 2g
- Sugars: 5.6g
- Protein: 3g
- Sodium: 5mg

CANTALOUPE YOGURT BOWL

Here's a refreshingly cool treat for those hot summer days. This is the best type of snack because of its endless possibilities! Prefer honeydew to cantaloupe? Cottage cheese to yogurt? Strawberries to blueberries? Want to add granola for texture and crunch? Want to add frozen yogurt for a summertime dessert? With a fruit bowl snack like this, the sky's the limit!

Prep to finish: 5 minutes
Difficulty: Easy
Yield: 2 servings
Serving Size: ½ cantaloupe; ¼ c. yogurt; 10 blueberries

Ingredients:
- 1 cantaloupe, cut in half
- ½ c. plain or vanilla low-fat yogurt (use Greek yogurt, if preferred)
- 20 fresh blueberries

Instructions:
1. Cut cantaloupe in half, using spoon scrape out insides to form 2 bowls.
2. Place ¼ c. yogurt into each cantaloupe half and top yogurt with 10 blueberries.
3. Serve immediately.

Nutritional info:
- Calories: 98
- Total Fat: 1.7g
- Total Carbohydrates: 14.1g
- Dietary Fiber: 0.6g
- Sugars: 2.8g
- Protein: 7g
- Sodium: 97mg

WATERMELON-FETA WEDGES

Here is yet another lip-smacking snack that is as refreshing as it is delicious. The combination will create an explosion of flavors in your mouth. These work brilliantly as appetizers for parties and entertaining, as well!

Prep to finish: 5 minutes
Difficulty: Easy
Yield: 8 servings
Serving Size: 3 wedges

Ingredients:
- 6 ounces of feta cheese
- ½ pound of watermelon
- Fresh basil leaves
- toothpicks

Instructions:
1. Slice feta into very thin 1" square slices (they should be at most a 1/8" thick) Note: 1-ounce of feta when sliced as instructed should produce 4 squares. By the time all the feta is cut, you should end up with 24 squares.
2. Now, cut the watermelon into 1" cubes.
3. Place one feta square on top of each watermelon cube. Place a basil leaf in the center of each feta slice.
4. Take a toothpick and push it through the center of the basil leaf, all the way through to the center of the watermelon cube, to hold all layers in place. Keep refrigerated until ready to use. May be prepared up to 4 hours in advance.
5. Serve cold. Serving size: 3 wedges.

Nutritional info:
- Calories: 66
- Total Fat: 4.5g
- Total Carbohydrates: 3g
- Dietary Fiber: 0g
- Sugars: 0.9g
- Protein: 1.1g
- Sodium: 79mg

FRUIT AND CHOCOLATE SNACK PLATE

This fruit and chocolate snack plate is a vitamin-packed antioxidant powerhouse. Not only does it contain anti-aging, healing, and weight loss inducing properties – it tastes delicious!

Prep to finish: 5 minutes
Difficulty: Easy
Yield: 2 servings
Serving Size: ½ of the plate

Ingredients:
- 2 small, ripe peaches – sliced
- ¼ c. fresh raspberries
- ¼ c. fresh blueberries
- 2 tbsp. semisweet mini chocolate chips - get dark chocolate for an even healthier choice!
- ½ tsp. ground cinnamon
- Pinch of nutmeg

Instructions:
1. Place sliced peaches in a bowl or sealable freezer bag. Sprinkle cinnamon and nutmeg over peaches and toss or shake to coat. Divide peaches and arrange on two separate serving plates.
2. Place 1/8 cup each of raspberries and blueberries alongside peaches on both plates.
3. Top each plate with 1 tbsp. chocolate chips.
4. Serve immediately.

Nutritional info:
- Calories: 98
- Total Fat: 3.2g
- Total Carbohydrates: 11g
- Dietary Fiber: 3.2g
- Sugars: 4.7g
- Protein: 6.7g
- Sodium: 118mg

CRANBERRY ORANGE PARFAIT

Dried cranberries, orange zest, vanilla-flavored Greek yogurt...the ingredients fit together perfectly. Every craving you could ever have will be knocked out by one bite of this healthful snack – whether you are in the mood for salty, sweet, sour, or umami– this snack's got your back!

Prep to finish: 5 minutes
Difficulty: Easy
Yield: 2 servings
Serving Size: 1 parfait

Ingredients:

- 2 c. vanilla-flavored Greek yogurt (may use plain, if preferred)
- 2 tsp. orange zest
- 1 tsp. vanilla bean scrapings
- 2 tsp. ground flaxseeds
- 2 oranges, peeled and sliced (enough to make 2 cups)
- 2 tbsp. dried cranberries
- 2 tbsp. unsalted chopped walnuts

Instructions:

1. Combine yogurt, orange zest, vanilla and flaxseeds in a bowl. Blend Well. Spoon ½ c. of the yogurt mixture into two parfait dishes.
2. Layer each parfait dish with ½ c. orange slices, ½ tbsp. cranberries, and ½ tbsp. walnuts.
3. Next, top each dish with another ½ c. yogurt, followed by ½ c. orange slices, ½ tbsp. cranberries, and ½ tbsp. walnuts. Serve immediately.

Nutritional info:
- Calories: 100
- Total Fat: 2.8g
- Total Carbohydrates: 17.3g
- Dietary Fiber: 0.7g
- Sugars: 14g
- Protein: 5g
- Sodium: 90mg

Recipes Under 250 Calories

Dessert Recipes

LOW-CALORIE S'MORES

Crunchy graham crackers, fluffy marshmallows, decadent drizzled chocolate – who ever thought eating healthy could be so good – and so much fun! Note: These are a quick and easy dessert, but they need a watchful eye when in the broiler – they can go from lightly toasted to black-ash burnt in a matter of seconds!

Prep to finish: 5 minutes
Difficulty: Easy
Yield: 2 servings
Serving Size: 2 s'mores squares

Ingredients:
- 2 whole graham crackers, broke in half along break line
- 4 medium-sized marshmallows
- 2 tbsp. semisweet chocolate chips, melted (may use dark chocolate chips, if preferred)

Instructions:
1. To begin, place oven rack in the upper-third of the oven; preheat broiler.
2. Prepare s'mores by placing the four graham cracker squares onto a baking sheet and topping each square with one marshmallow.
3. Melt chocolate chips in microwave, to do so, heat at 80% power for 30 seconds and then in 10 to 15 second intervals until completely melted.
4. Place baking sheet in broiler and broil for about 30 to 40 seconds with the oven door ajar. Watch constantly until the marshmallows are golden brown.
5. Remove s'mores from oven. Immediately drizzle each s'more with melted chocolate.
6. Place 2 s'mores onto a serving plate and serve immediately.

Nutritional info:
- Calories: 98
- Total Fat: 3g
- Total Carbohydrates: 18g
- Dietary Fiber: 3.7g
- Sugars: 8.3g
- Protein: 1g
- Sodium: 70mg

MINI CHEESECAKES

Tiny, yet filling and delicious – finally, here's a lip-smacking cheesecake that's under 90 calories per serving! Creamy filling on a villa wafer crust, this is one dessert that will have you jumping for joy! Note: These can be frozen and pulled out for any party, special occasion, after-dinner dessert, or midnight snack.

Prep to finish: Prep time - 10 minutes; Cook time: 10-12 minutes; Total time – 20 to 22 minutes
Difficulty: Easy
Yield: 15 servings (*makes 30 cheesecakes)*
Serving Size: 2 mini cheesecakes

Ingredients:
- 2 c. graham crackers, crushed
- 1/8 c. granulated sugar
- ¼ c. butter or margarine, melted
- 16 ounces Neufchatel cheese
- *1 cup nonfat or 1% cottage cheese (no salt added)
- 2 large eggs
- ¼ c. granulated sugar
- 1 tsp. vanilla bean scrapings
- Fresh strawberries and blueberries (optional.)
- 30 muffin liners

Instructions:
1. Begin by preheating oven to 325°F. Place oven rack in to the center of the oven.
2. Take out your 12 cup muffin pan and place a liner in each cup.
3. In a medium-sized mixing bowl prepare the graham cracker crust by combining the crushed graham crackers, 1/8 c. sugar, and ¼ c. melted butter or margarine. Stir until well blended and evenly coated with melted butter.
4. Press 1 tsp. graham cracker crust into the bottom of each liner, until the bottom of the liner is covered.
5. In a medium-size mixing bowl, combine Neufchatel cheese, cottage cheese, eggs, sugar, and vanilla bean scrapings. Using an electric mixer, blend until smooth and creamy.
6. When the filling is ready, place 2 tbsp. of filling over the crust in each muffin liner.
7. Place muffin pan in oven and bake 10 to 12 minutes or until the filling becomes firm in the center. Remove from oven and cool completely, then chill.
8. Serve either chilled or at room temp. To serve, place 2 mini cheesecakes onto a serving dish and garnish each cake with a few blueberries and/or sliced strawberries.

For one mini cheesecake without berries: 87 calories, 5.0 g fat, 7.1 g carbohydrates, 5.4 g sugar, 3.6 g protein, 0 g fiber, 113 mg sodium, 2 PointsPlus

Nutritional info:
- Calories: 194
- Total Fat: 10.7g
- Total Carbohydrates: 16.2
- Dietary Fiber: 0.8g
- Sugars: 12.8g
- Protein: 7.2g
- Sodium: 226mg

Tiramisu Parfait

If you're a fan of the classic, you will appreciate this lighter, low-calorie, healthier parfait spin-off of the original. Tiramisu offers a timeless, enchanting, and memorable taste that will turn you into a tiramisu aficionado for life! They may take more time than other desserts, but once you take that first bite - you will be so happy you took the time!

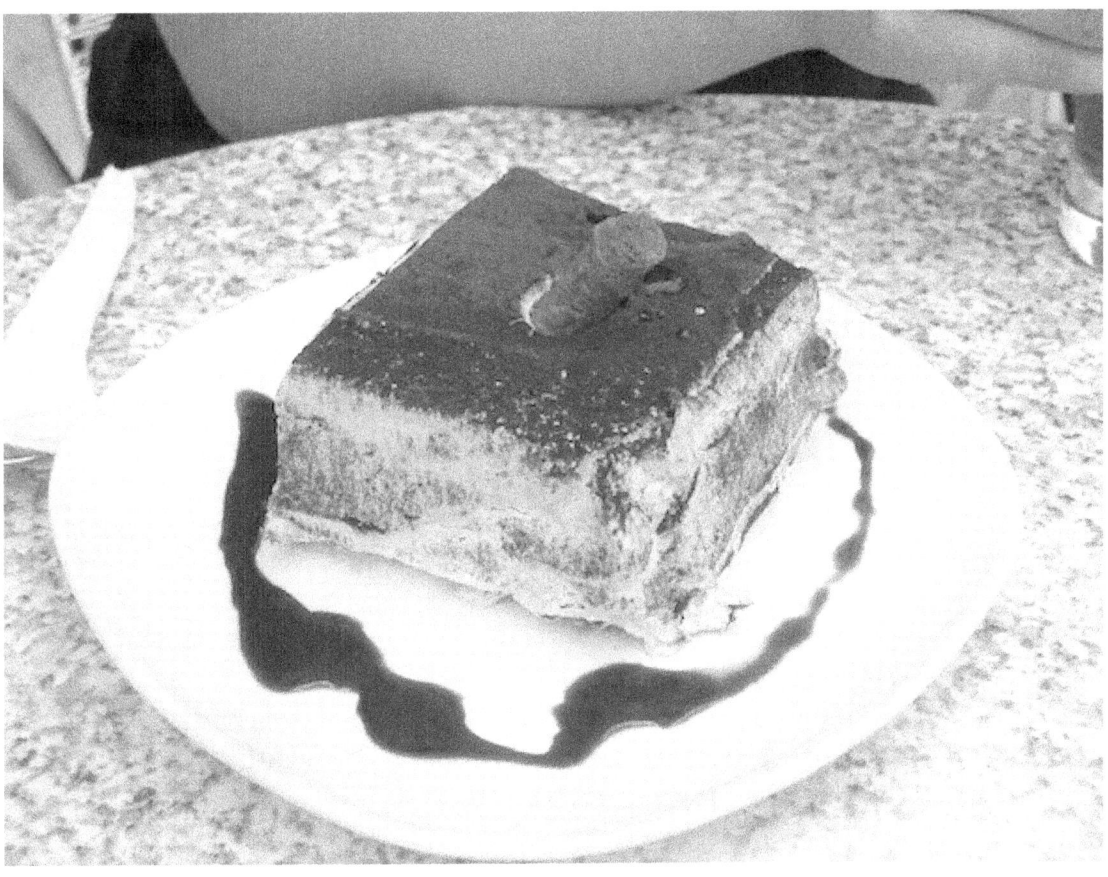

Prep to finish: Prep time – 40 minutes; Chill time – 8 hours; Total time – 8 hours 40 minutes
Difficulty: Easy
Yield: 2 servings
Serving Size: 1

Ingredients:
- 1 ½ tsp. instant coffee granules
- 1 ¾ tbsp. boiling water
- 2/3 c. cold nonfat milk
- 1/2 to 1 package sugar-free instant vanilla pudding mix
- 1 1/3-ounces fat-free plain cream cheese
- 1/2 package ladyfinger cookies, split and cubed
- 1 cup fat-free whipped topping

- 2 tbsp. semisweet miniature chocolate chips
- 1 tsp. baking cocoa
- 2 parfait dishes

Instructions:

1. Begin by placing coffee granules in small bowl and pouring 1 ¾ tbsp. boiling water over the granules, stir the coffee granules until they are completely dissolved in the boiling water. Set aside and cool to room temperature.
2. Meanwhile, place the pudding mix and cold milk in medium-sized mixing bowl and whisk together for 2 minutes. Let stand for 2 more minutes or until the pudding becomes soft-set.
3. In a separate medium-sized mixing bowl, beat cream cheese with electric mixer until smooth. Then gradually fold the cream cheese into the pudding mixture. Blend well.
4. Next, place the cubed ladyfingers in a bowl, add the now room-temp coffee and very gently toss to coat the ladyfingers with coffee. Let stand for 5 minutes in order for the ladyfingers to really soak in the coffee.
5. Take out two parfait dishes. Place the ingredients into the parfait dishes in the following order:
   - First Layer:
     - ¼ of the cubed ladyfingers into the bottom of each parfait dish, followed by
     - ¼ of the cream cheese-pudding mixture, followed by
     - ¼ c. whipped topping, followed by
     - ½ tbsp. chocolate chips
   - Second Layer:
     - ¼ of the cubed ladyfingers into the bottom of each parfait dish, followed by
     - ¼ of the cream cheese-pudding mixture, followed by
     - ¼ c. whipped topping, followed by
     - ½ tbsp. chocolate chips
6. Place both parfaits in the refrigerator to chill for 8 hours.
7. Before serving, dust the tops of the parfaits with cocoa powder.

Nutritional info:
- Calories: 189
- Total Fat: 3g
- Total Carbohydrates: 32g
- Dietary Fiber: 1g
- Sugars: 9.8g
- Protein: 7g
- Sodium: 373mg

MINI MOLTEN CHOCOLATE CAKES WITH HOT CHOCOLATE SAUCE

Ready for a real treat that will taste so good, it will feel like you're breaking all the rules? Ready for gooey, moist, chocolate cake doused in a warm and decadent chocolate sauce? Ready for not only one of these mini pieces of heaven – but 2 of them?! Brace yourself! With this mouthwatering dessert you not only get one cake for 244 calories – the serving size is 2 cakes!!!

Prep to finish: Prep time: 10 minutes; Cook time: 10 minutes; Total time: 20 minutes
Difficulty: Medium
Yield: 6 servings
Serving Size: 2 cakes

Ingredients:
- 20 tablespoons (2½ sticks) butter
- 2 c. (16 ounces) semisweet chocolate chips
- 1 c. all-purpose flour
- 3 c. confectioners' (powdered) sugar
- 6 large eggs
- 6 egg yolks
- 2 teaspoon vanilla bean scrapings
- 1 tsp. instant coffee powder (optional)
- Powdered sugar for dusting (optional)
- Fresh raspberries to garnish (optional)

- (12) 6 ounce custard cups (ramekin cups) or (1) 12 cup muffin pan
- Nonstick cooking spray

Instructions:
1. Preheat oven to 425° F.
2. Spray each custard cup or the 12 cup muffin pan with non-stick cooking spray.
3. In a medium-sized microwaveable mixing bowl, combine chocolate chips and butter. Place bowl in the microwave and heat for 60 seconds at 50% power, then continue microwaving in 30-second intervals until butter and chocolate chips are completely melted and form a smooth and creamy consistency.
4. Stir the flour and sugar into the chocolate-butter sauce and stir until fairly well blended.
5. Next, add the eggs and the egg yolks to the butter-chocolate mixture and stir with spoon or use an electric mixer until the ingredients are well blended.
6. Next stir in the vanilla and instant coffee and stir until all ingredients are well combined.
7. Place an even amount of batter into each custard cup or muffin pan cup. If using custard cups, place the cups on top of a baking sheet.
8. Place the baking sheet or muffin pan into the oven and bake for about 10 minutes, or until the edges of each cake are firm but the center is runny.
9. Run a knife around the edge to loosen and drop onto a serving dish.

10. Dust each cake with powdered sugar and garnish with a couple fresh raspberries, if desired.

Nutritional info:
- Calories: 244
- Total Fat: 17g
- Total Carbohydrates: 27g
- Dietary Fiber: 2g
- Sugars: 8.7g
- Protein: 3g
- Sodium: 64mg

Coconut Macaroons Drizzled with Dark Chocolate

Treat yourself with a delicate and unforgettable coconut macaroon that is drizzled in melted dark chocolate and garnished with Fleur de Sel – a form of sea salt.

Prep to finish: Prep time: 15 minutes; Cook time: 15 minutes; Total time: 30 minutes
Difficulty: Easy
Yield: 8 servings
Serving Size: 2 macaroons

Ingredients:
- ½ cup sugar
- ¼ cup water
- ¼ cup Asian coconut milk (full fat version)
- ¼ tsp. kosher salt
- 2 cups unsweetened desiccated coconut
- 1 egg white (approx. 3 tablespoons)
- ¼ cup dark chocolate chips
- ½ tsp. Fleur de Sel (optional)

Instructions:
1. To begin, preheat oven to 350° F.
2. Place a non-stick pan over medium heat and add in sugar, water, coconut milk, and salt. Heat until the mixture comes to a medium simmer. Continue cooking for 5 minutes. The mixture should appear whitish in color, bubbly, and a little bit thinner than maple syrup, but thicker than water.
3. Next, Place 1½ c. of flaked coconut in a medium-sized mixing bowl. Gradually stir the warm sugar water mixture into the coconut and stir until the flaked coconut is well coated.
4. Stir in the egg white and then the remaining flaked coconut. Continue stirring until well mixed.
5. Pack an ice cream or cookie scoop firmly with the coconut mixture and drop macaroons on a parchment paper-lined baking sheet. Place macaroons 2-inches apart.
6. Place in oven and bake for 13 to 15 minutes or until the outer shell is golden brown and crispy to the touch.
7. Remove the baking sheet from oven and allow the macaroons to cool on the baking sheet for approximately 30 minutes.
8. Meanwhile, prepare the dark chocolate drizzle by melting the chocolate chips in the microwave for 30 seconds and then in 15 second intervals, stirring in between intervals, until all chips are melted and the chocolate is smooth and runny enough to drizzle.
9. Finally drizzle dark chocolate over the tops of the macaroons and garnish each with a few sprinkles of Fleur de Sel.

Nutritional info:
- Calories: 97

- Total Fat: 3g
- Total Carbohydrates: 17.4g
- Dietary Fiber: 0.4g
- Sugars: 17g
- Protein: 1g
- Sodium: 59mg

Recipes Under 300 Calories

Dinner Recipes

PARMESAN-CRUSTED TILAPIA

Curb your seafood cravings with this mouthwatering tilapia coated with a crunchy parmesan crust and baked to perfection. A light texture and bursting with flavor, this versatile fish is low in saturated fat and calories, but still is quick to fill the tummy and keep you smiling! Tilapia is perfect for the weight loss dieter. It is the ideal fish to bake, grill, fry, or broil and can be prepared in many different ways using a variety of ingredients – explore all of the wonderful tilapia recipes online that will keep your taste buds happy on both feed and fast days!

Prep to finish: Prep time - 10 minutes; Total time – 25 minutes
Difficulty: Easy
Yield: 2 servings
Serving Size: (1) 5-ounce tilapia fillet

Ingredients:
- 1/3 c. parmesan cheese, grated
- 1 ½ tbsp. extra virgin olive oil
- 3/4 lime yields lime juice
- (2) 5-ounce tilapia fillets
- Pinch of preferred seasoning

Directions:
1. Preheat oven to 450°F.
2. Rinse and pat dry each tilapia fillet with a paper towel. Sprinkle each fillet with preferred seasoning.
3. Place fillets in a glass baking dish, and bake for approximately 5 minutes. Meanwhile, in a shallow bowl combine lime juice and olive oil.
4. Remove fish from oven. Turn on broiler.
5. Coat each fillet with lemon/olive oil mixture and dip into grated parmesan to form a crust.
6. Place fillets under broiler for about 1 ½-2 minutes or until the fish begins to brown along the edges. Remove fish from broiler and transfer each fillet to a serving dish. Serve immediately.

Nutritional info:
- Calories: 203
- Total Fat: 13.4g
- Total Carbohydrates: 1.5g
- Dietary Fiber: 0.1g

- Sugars: 0.31g
- Protein: 19.5g
- Sodium: 208mg

SHRIMP TACOS WITH YOGURT SAUCE

Shrimp tacos are perfect for hot summer days or for any time of the year – and anytime of the day! Cool, fresh, deliciously crisp fillings that are low-calorie and taste excellent. This is a refreshing protein-packed dish that makes eating healthy a WHOLE LOTTA FUN!

Prep to finish: Prep time - 15 minutes; Cook time – 10 minutes; Total time – 25 minutes
Difficulty: Easy
Yield: 2 servings
Serving Size: 2 tacos

Ingredients:
- Olive oil cooking spray
- 2 tbsp. salsa
- 4 whole-wheat tortillas
- 1 ½ limes juiced
- 1 lime, peel intact – cut into wedges
- 6 ounces small shrimp – tail on, fully cooked
- ½ c. plain Greek yogurt
- ¼ tbsp. plus 1 tsp. dried cumin
- ¼ tsp. ground oregano
- ½ tbsp. cayenne pepper
- ¼ ounce dill
- 2 c. cabbage, shredded
- ½ c. fresh cilantro, torn or chopped
- 1 clove garlic, minced
- 1/8 c. any preferred low-calorie mayonnaise

Instructions:
1. In a skillet, coated with olive oil cooking spray, sauté shrimp for 2 minutes over medium to medium-high heat.
2. Add in fresh minced garlic, 1 tsp. dried cumin, 1 tbsp. salsa, and the juice from 1 lime.
3. Prepare the yogurt sauce: In a medium-sized mixing bowl combine yogurt, mayo, oregano, remaining cumin, dill, and cayenne pepper.
4. Prepare cilantro, lime, and cabbage as directed.
5. Warm tortillas in the microwave or oven. Fill warm tortillas with sautéed shrimp, shredded cabbage, fresh cilantro, and ¼ of the yogurt sauce. Serve alongside 2 tbsp. salsa and a couple of lime wedges. Serving size is 2 tacos.

Nutritional info:
- Calories: 247
- Total Fat: 5.7g
- Total Carbohydrates: 34.2g

- Dietary Fiber: 4.5g
- Sugars: 7.2g
- Protein: 11.1g
- Sodium: 655mg

EGGPLANT LASAGNA

Tender crisp eggplant nestled among hot and bubbly mozzarella cheese and a magnificent cottage-cheese sauce makes this lasagna dish a rich experience and a joy to eat, yet leaves you feeling guilt-free. Try adding black olives, other veggies, different cheeses, or your favorite ingredients to change up the recipe and better meet your personal taste!

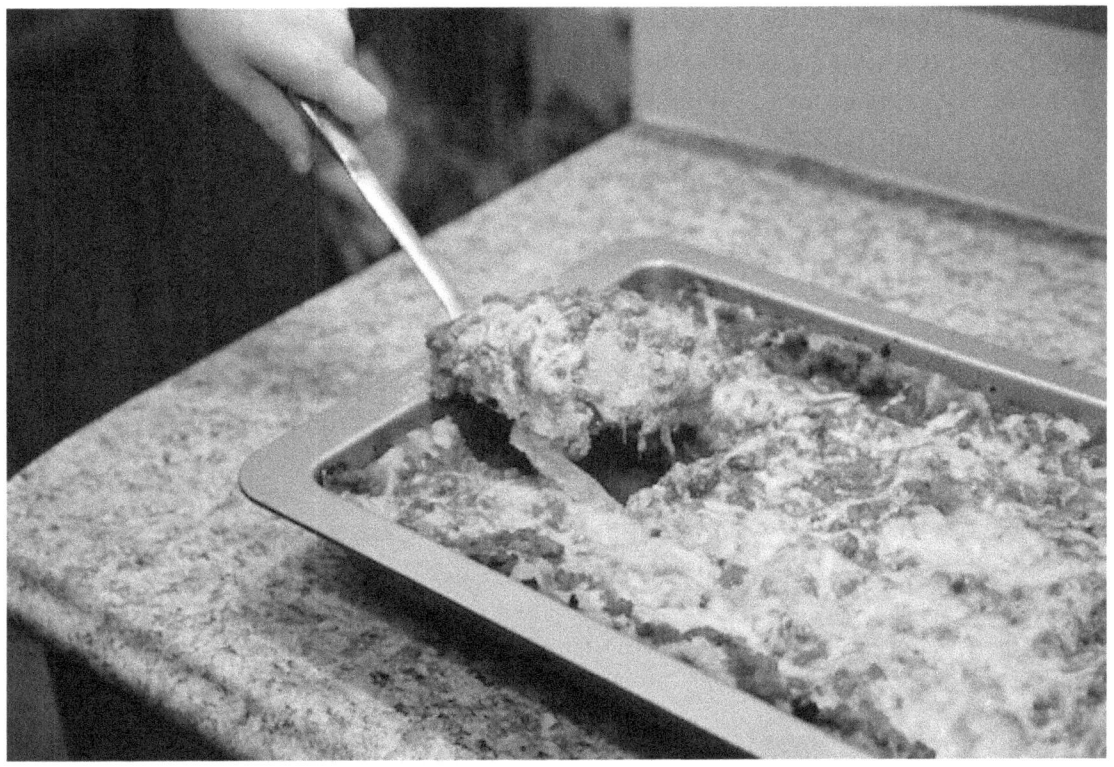

Prep to finish: 5 minutes
Difficulty: Easy
Yield: 2 servings
Serving Size: Half of the lasagna

Ingredients:
- 1 c. low-fat mozzarella cheese, grated
- 3 tbsp. parmesan cheese
- 1 medium egg
- ½ tsp. nutmeg
- 6 basil leaves
- 1 ½ c. marinara sauce
- ½ eggplant
- 1 c. low fat cottage cheese

- Olive oil spray
- 1/8 tsp. sea salt
- 1/8 tsp. fresh ground black pepper

Instructions:

1. Preheat oven to 400 °F.
2. Prepare the eggplant. If you prefer the eggplant peeled, do so now. Slice the eggplant thinly into rounds. Lay the slices on a paper towel and sprinkle a pinch of salt over the eggplant - this will help to absorb any extra liquid.
3. Spread the eggplant pieces onto a cookie sheet that has been coated in olive oil spray. Spray the eggplant pieces evenly with the spray as well. Bake the eggplant for approximately 5 minutes or until the eggplant reaches desired crispiness or tenderness. Remove eggplant from oven and set aside.
4. Prepare cheese mixture: in a medium-sized mixing bowl, combine 2 tbsp. parmesan, salt, pepper, nutmeg, and one whole egg. An electric mixer works wonders towards achieving a smooth consistency.
5. Spread a thin layer of sauce across the bottom of an 8x8 or smaller square baking dish. Begin layering eggplant, cheese mixture, and all but 1/8 cup of the shredded mozzarella.
6. Finally, pour marinara sauce over the top of the lasagna and sprinkle with the remaining mozzarella and parmesan cheeses.
7. Bake in oven for 20 to 25 minutes, until cheese is melted, bubbly, and the layers are heated through. Divide lasagna in half and transfer to serving dish. Eat hot.

Nutritional info:
- Calories: 209
- Total Fat: 8.8g
- Total Carbohydrates: 21.1g
- Dietary Fiber: 3.7g
- Sugars: 14.6g
- Protein: 13.5g
- Sodium: 354mg

GRILLED SALMON WITH CREAMY COCONUT GLAZE

Get ready for the taste of a true island dinner! You will really feel as if you are in the middle of a tropical paradise while savoring every last bite. This amazing take on salmon is easy and fast to prepare and loaded with nutritional goodness!!!

Prep to finish: 18 minutes
Difficulty: Easy
Yield: 2 servings
Serving Size: (1) salmon filet and ¼ c. coconut glaze

Ingredients:
- (2) 5- to 6-ounce salmon fillets (wild caught)
- ¼ tsp. sea salt (opt)
- ¼ tsp. freshly ground black pepper
- 2 tsp. coconut oil
- 1 large shallot, diced
- 3 cloves garlic, minced
- Zest of one lemon
- Juice of one lemon
- ½ c. coconut milk
- 2 tbsp. fresh basil, chopped

Instructions:
1. Preheat oven to 350°F.
2. Place salmon in a shallow baking dish and season each side of the salmon fillet with sea salt and fresh ground black pepper.
3. Place a medium-sized sauté pan over medium heat. When the pan becomes hot, add the coconut oil, garlic, and shallots. Sauté for about 3 minutes or until the shallots become tender and the garlic fragrant.
4. Next, add in the lemon zest, lemon juice, and coconut milk. Bring the contents to a low boil. Reduce heat to low and add the basil. Blend the ingredients together thoroughly.
5. Pour the coconut glaze over the salmon and place the salmon in the oven to bake, uncovered, for approximately 10 minutes, or until salmon has reached your desired temperature and doneness.
6. Remove the salmon fillets from the oven. Transfer each to a separate serving dish. Drizzle any remaining coconut glaze left behind in the baking dish over the top of the salmon fillets. Serve immediately.

Nutritional info:
- Calories: 206
- Total Fat: 8.3g
- Total Carbohydrates: 8.6g

- Dietary Fiber: 1.2g
- Sugars: 4.8g
- Protein: 15.4g
- Sodium: 190mg

ALOHA CHICKEN KABOBS

If you like grilled chicken and you love skewers, your heart will skip a beat when you taste these heavenly chicken kabobs. The grilled chicken glaze has a tropical-honey flavor that is out of this world and under 250 calories! String your favorite fruits, veggies, and other ingredients on the skewers for scrumptious mealtime fun!

Prep to finish: 20 minutes
Difficulty: Easy
Yield: 2 serving
Serving Size: 3 skewers

Ingredients:

- 3 tbsp. reduced sodium soy sauce
- 3 tbsp. brown raw cane sugar
- 2 tbsp. sherry
- 1 tbsp. sesame oil
- ¼ tsp. ground ginger
- ¼ tsp. garlic powder
- ¼ tsp. organic honey
- 3 skinless, boneless chicken breast halves - cut into 2-inch pieces
- (1) 20 ounce can pineapple chunks in juice, drained
- Skewers (soak wooden skewers in water before using)
- High-heat cooking spray

Instructions:

1. In a shallow glass dish, mix the soy sauce, brown raw cane sugar, sherry, sesame oil, ginger, and garlic powder.
2. Stir the chicken pieces and pineapple into the marinade until well coated.
3. Preheat grill to medium-high heat.
4. Lightly oil the grill grate. Thread chicken and pineapple alternately onto skewers.
5. Grill 5 to 7 minutes, turning occasionally, or until juices run clear. Place 3 skewers onto a serving plate and enjoy!

Nutritional info:
- Calories 225:
- Total Fat: 6.8g
- Total Carbohydrates: 9.4g
- Dietary Fiber: 1.7g
- Sugars: 5.2g
- Protein: 28.9g
- Sodium: 272mg

CRAB-STUFFED PORTOBELLO MUSHROOMS

This is a delicious and fun protein-rich dish that is easy to prepare and quick to make. The combination of fresh baby spinach, onion, tender mushrooms, and flavorful crab meat make this a meal to remember and one that you will want to prepare again and again!

Prep to finish: 20 minutes
Difficulty: Easy
Yield: 2 servings
Serving Size: 3 medium-sized or 2 large-sized stuffed mushroom caps

Ingredients:

- 1 to 2 c. (8 ounces) cooked crab meat
- 1 tbsp. plus 1/2 tbsp. extra-virgin olive oil
- 2 c. fresh baby spinach, chopped
- 4 to 6 medium- to large-sized Portobello mushrooms (large enough to be stuffed)
- 1/8 c. white onions, chopped fine
- 1 cloves garlic, minced (or 1 tsp. pre-minced garlic)
- 1/4 tsp. dried basil, crushed
- 1/4 tsp. dried oregano, crushed
- 1/8 tsp. ground ginger
- 1 oz. apple cider
- 1 tbsp. fresh-squeezed lemon juice

Instructions:

1. Preheat oven to 425°F.
2. Heat 1 tbsp. olive oil in a sauté pan over medium heat. Once the oil is hot, add the spinach and cook for about 3 minutes or until the spinach begins to wilt slightly.
3. If the Portobello mushrooms have stems, remove them. Cut off the top of each mushroom and set the tops aside. Using a spoon, carve out some of the insides of each mushroom.
4. Take the stem from each mushroom and chop them up. Place the chopped stems in a skillet over medium heat (you can also place the carved insides from each mushroom in the skillet as well). Also add the onion, garlic, apple cider, and lemon juice. Cook for 2 to 3 minutes or until onion becomes slightly tender.
5. Add the cooked spinach to the skillet. Reduce the heat to low and cook for about 2 minutes to evaporate any liquid remaining from the spinach. Stir in the basil, oregano, and ginger. Blend contents together thoroughly.
6. Add the crab meat to the spinach mixture and stir until mixed well throughout the mixture. Cook for 3 to 4 minutes or until crab is heated through.
7. Place mushrooms into a baking dish and spoon some of the crab mixture into each of the mushrooms. Brush 1/4 tbsp. of olive oil over the top and sides of each mushroom. Place in the oven and bake for 8 to 10 minutes or until the mushrooms are tender. Remove mushrooms from oven and divide onto two separate serving plates. Serve immediately.

Nutritional info:
- Calories: 266
- Total Fat: 12g
- Total Carbohydrates: 13g
- Dietary Fiber: 3g
- Sugars: 5g
- Protein: 28g
- Sodium: 408mg

Recipes Under 400 Calories

Soup and Salad Recipes

CHIPOTLE CHICKEN CHOWDER

A creamy, thick, chipotle-spiced chowder with chicken, peppers, and just the right amount of seasoning to keep you full and satisfied on fast days and everyday!

Prep to finish: Prep time - 5 minutes; Cook time – 20 minutes; Total time: 25 minutes.
Difficulty: Easy
Yield: 4 servings
Serving Size: 1 cup of soup

Ingredients:
- 12 ounces evaporated milk, nonfat
- 1 tsp. cumin
- 1 tbsp. extra virgin olive oil
- 8 ounces chicken breast meat, chopped
- 14 ounces reduced sodium chicken broth
- ¾ c. chopped onions
- ¾ c. chopped green peppers
- ¾ c. chopped red peppers
- 2 chipotle peppers in adobo sauce
- 4 fluid-ounce water
- 3 tbsp. cornstarch

Instructions:
1. Add the olive oil to a large saucepan and place over medium heat.
2. Once the oil is hot, add in green and red peppers, chopped onion, and cumin. Cook for about 3 minutes, stirring occasionally.
3. Slowly stir in chicken broth, water, and chipotle peppers. Bring to a boil.
4. Reduce heat; simmer, covered, for approximately 8 minutes. Stir in chicken breast.
5. Place the cornstarch into a small bowl and gradually stir in 1/3 cup of the milk. Once cornstarch mixture is well blended, slowly add to the broth in the saucepan.
6. Finally, add in the remaining milk. Continue to cook over medium heat, stirring frequently, until soup is thick and bubbly.
7. Transfer to soup bowl and garnish with sliced green onions, if desired.

Nutritional info:
- Calories: 229
- Total Fat: 4.6g

- Total Carbohydrates: 24g
- Dietary Fiber: 1.8g
- Sugars: 13.2g
- Protein: 21.8g
- Sodium: 268mg

SHRIMP STEW

This delicious shrimp stew is perfect for cold days, or chilly summer evenings. You'll feel like you are in New Orleans, with these gumbo inspired flavors!

Prep to finish: Prep time -10 minutes; Cook time – 20 minutes; Total time – 30 minutes
Difficulty: Easy
Yield: 4 servings
Serving Size: 1 cup

Ingredients:
- 1 ¾ c. low-sodium chicken broth
- 2 links Italian chicken and beef sausage
- 8 ounces shrimp, fully cooked
- 1 tbsp. olive oil
- 2 medium carrots peeled & sliced thin
- 2 cloves garlic
- 1 c. sliced onion
- ½ c. fresh parsley
- 1 c. diced potato
- 1/8 c. flour
- Salt and pepper, to taste
- 1 c. water

Instructions:
1. Begin by heating oil in a Dutch oven or large saucepan over medium heat.
2. Once oil is hot, add potato, carrot, garlic, onion, and sausage.
3. Season with salt and pepper, and cook for about 15 minutes or until potatoes are tender-crisp, stirring occasionally.
4. Sprinkle the flour over the vegetables. Stir in broth and one cup of water. Bring to a boil.
5. Reduce heat and simmer. Cook for approximately 5 minutes or until potatoes are cooked through.
6. Add shrimp to soup. Cover and simmer for 3 to 4 minutes or until shrimp are warmed through.
7. Transfer one cup of soup to serving bowl. Garnish with parsley (optional) and enjoy!

Nutritional info:
- Calories: 278
- Total Fat: 14g
- Total Carbohydrates: 17g
- Dietary Fiber: 3g
- Sugars: 3g
- Protein: 23g
- Sodium: 553mg

FIRE ROASTED TOMATO AND SWEET POTATO CHILI

Sweet potatoes, fire roasted tomatoes, and the perfect combination of seasonings makes this an award-winning chili worthy of a first-place ribbon!

Prep to finish: Prep time: 20 minutes; Cook time: 20 minutes; Total time: 40 minutes
Difficulty: Easy
Yield: 6 servings
Serving Size: 1 cup

Ingredients:
- ½ c. fire roasted crushed tomatoes
- 1 ½ c. chunky tomato sauce
- 1 c. dark red kidney beans
- 4 c. vegetable broth
- 6 tsp. garlic
- 4 tbsp. chili powder
- 1 tbsp. cumin
- 2 tsp. ground oregano
- 1 tbsp. olive oil
- 2 medium carrots, sliced
- 1 ounce onion, diced
- 1 5" long sweet potato, chopped into chunks
- 1 small red pepper, diced or cut into 1" strips
- 1 large yellow pepper, diced or cut into 1" strips
- 12 ounces cooked kidney beans

Instructions:
1. Begin by cleaning and preparing all vegetables as directed above.
2. Add oil to a sauté pan and place over medium-high heat.
3. When oil is hot and glistening, sauté all veggies beginning with sweet potatoes, followed by carrots, onions, and garlic for 7 minutes.
4. Add peppers and cook for an additional 7 to 10 minutes.
5. Add tomatoes, followed by the rest of the seasonings. Simmer for 5 minutes.
6. Finally add vegetable broth and kidney beans and bring to a boil.
7. Reduce heat and simmer for 20 minutes.
8. Transfer one cup to a serving bowl and add salt and pepper, to taste.

Nutritional info:
- Calories: 203
- Total Fat: 4.1g
- Total Carbohydrates: 38.1g
- Dietary Fiber: 38.1g

- Sugars: 10.4g
- Protein: 8.7g
- Sodium: 742mg

VEGGIE BEEF SOUP

This soup is perfect for cold afternoons or for those days where you are just feeling under the weather. Hot soup to warm your tummy and take your cares away! There really is something magical about a bowl of warm soup on a cold day!

Prep to finish: Prep time: 15 minutes; Cook time: 60 minutes; Total time: 1 hour 15 minutes
Difficulty: Medium
Yield: 4 servings
Serving Size: 1 cup soup

Ingredients:
- 1 2/3 c. low sodium chicken broth
- 1 c. uncooked brown rice
- ¾ tsp. allspice
- ¾ tbsp. smoked paprika
- 1 ¼ tsp. fresh ground black pepper
- Sea salt, to taste
- 1/3 cup ground lean turkey
- 2 1/3 c. Savoy cabbage, shredded
- 1 to 2 medium carrots, sliced or diced
- 1 ¼ cloves garlic, diced
- 1/3 medium onion, diced
- 1/3 pound ground beef
- 1 c. tomato sauce
- 3 tbsp. extra virgin olive oil

Directions:
1. Begin by washing all veggies and preparing as directed above.]
2. Place a sauté pan over medium-high heat and add oil.
3. Once oil is hot and glistening, add onion, garlic and carrot and sauté for 3 to 5 minutes or until onion is translucent, garlic is fragrant, and all is tender.
4. Now, add ground turkey AND beef. Cook for 10 to 12 minutes, or until both meats are just barely cooked through. Sprinkle on smoked paprika, allspice, sea salt, and black pepper.
5. Next, add the shredded cabbage and cook until it becomes wilted. Once cabbage is wilted, stir in tomato sauce and chicken stock.
6. If needed, add more sea salt and pepper, to taste. Continue cooking soup for about 30 more minutes in order to allow the cabbage to cook all the way through and so as to blend all the flavors.
7. While the soup is cooking, prepare brown rice according to package directions.
8. Once both soup and rice are finished cooking. Transfer one cup of soup to a soup bowl and top with ¼ cup brown rice. Eat immediately!

Nutritional info:
- Calories: 383
- Total Fat: 15g
- Total Carbohydrates: 48g
- Dietary Fiber: 5g
- Sugars: 6g
- Protein: 16g
- Sodium: 417mg

BARLEY AND MUSHROOM SOUP

This soup is a vegetarian delight. Plump, tender mushrooms, wholesome barley, tender carrots, celery, and onions and more create a soup that overflows with nutritional goodness and impeccable taste.

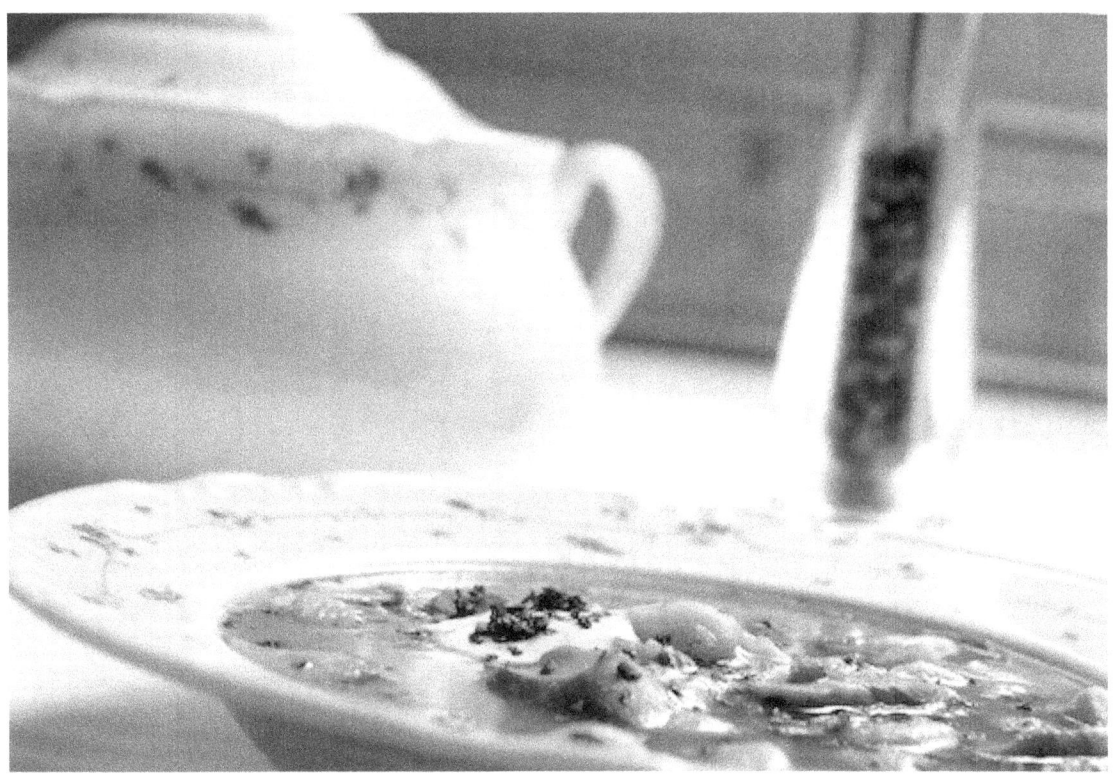

Prep to finish: Prep time: 20 minutes; Cook time: 45 minutes; Total time: 1 hour and 5 minutes
Difficulty: Easy
Yield: 6 servings
Serving Size: One cup soup

Ingredients:
- 1 dash fresh ground black pepper
- ½ tsp. thyme
- 1 dash salt
- 3 cups vegetable broth
- 1 cup chopped carrots
- 1 cup chopped celery
- 6 cloves garlic
- 3 cups pieces or slices mushrooms
- 1 cup chopped onions
- 2 large red potatoes
- 1/3 cup barley

Instructions:

1. Begin by washing and preparing all vegetables as directed.
2. Place a large pot or Dutch oven over medium-high to high heat.
3. Combine all ingredients in the order listed. Bring to a boil.
4. Reduce heat and simmer. Cover and continue cooking for 35 to 45 minutes or until all vegetables have reached desired tenderness.
5. Transfer one cup of soup to a bowl.
6. Serve immediately.

Nutritional info:
- Calories: 243
- Total Fat: 2.5g
- Total Carbohydrates: 48.2g
- Dietary Fiber: 7.1g
- Sugars: 6.4g
- Protein: 8.2g
- Sodium: 582mg

PASTA VEGGIE SALAD

Finally, a pasta salad that is healthy, low-calorie, quick and simple to make that will have your taste buds doing cartwheels. Try whipping up a big batch for parties and barbeques – this salad is sure to be a crowd pleaser!

Prep to finish: Prep time: 5 minutes; Cook time: 7 – 10 minutes (pasta); Total time: 1 hour (chill) 15 minutes
Difficulty: Easy
Yield: 2 servings
Serving Size: 1 1/2 cups pasta salad

Ingredients:
- 1 ½ c. penne rigate
- 2 tbsp. apple cider vinegar
- 1 large whole tomato, cut into wedges
- 2 tsp. leaves basil, chopped
- 1 stalk broccoli, cut into chunks or left whole.
- 1 large cucumber, sliced
- 3 large mushrooms, sliced
- 1 large yellow sweet pepper, chopped
- sea salt, to taste
- Fresh ground black pepper, to taste
- 1 tbsp. olive oil

Instructions:
1. Begin by cooking pasta as directed on package. Add salt to water to prevent the pasta from sticking. Boil pasta until al dente and then drain, rinse well with cool water, and set aside.
2. Wash and prepare all vegetables as directed above.
3. Prepare broccoli by blanching. Place in hot boiling water and let steam for 2 to 3 minutes or until broccoli is bright green. Then immediately plunge into ice water. This will maintain the bright green color.
4. Place cooked pasta and prepared vegetables in large mixing bowl. Mix in oil, vinegar, and remaining seasonings. Toss to coat pasta and vegetable with oil, vinegar, and seasonings.
5. Mix in oil, vinegar, and seasonings. Place in refrigerator and let chill for a minimum of 1 hour.
6. Place 1 cup pasta on salad plate and serve cold.

Nutritional info:
- Calories: 242
- Total Fat: 6g
- Total Carbohydrates: 40g

- Dietary Fiber: 5g
- Sugars: 4.1g
- Protein: 8.6g
- Sodium: 76mg

ZUCCHINI AVOCADO CARPACCIO

A light and refreshingly cool salad for a warm spring or hot summer day. Crisp zucchini and sweet avocado help to make this salad memorable and delicious.

Prep to finish: Prep time: 15 minutes
Difficulty: Easy
Yield: 2 servings
Serving Size: 2 cups salad

Ingredients:
- 1 tbsp. extra virgin olive oil
- ½ ripe avocado, thinly sliced
- 1 lemon for: 1 tbsp. fresh lemon juice; ¼ tsp. grated lemon zest
- 1 large zucchini, thinly sliced.
- ¼ cup sliced salted roasted almonds, chopped
- freshly ground black pepper, to taste
- sea salt, to taste

Instructions:
1. Begin by preparing the lemon. Peel place 1 tbsp. juice into a small bowl. Grate peel and place1/4 tsp. lemon zest into bowl with lemon juice.

2. Using whisk, stir the olive oil into lemon juice mixture. Stir in sea salt and black pepper to taste.

3. Using a sharp knife, slice the zucchini into razor-thin slices. Repeat with avocado.

4. On a salad plate combine overlapping layers of zucchini and avocado slices. Drizzle lemon-olive oil dressing mixture all over the surface of the salad. Top off with 1/8 c. sliced almonds on each salad.

5. Enjoy!

Nutritional info:
- Calories: 213
- Total Fat: 17.7g
- Total Carbohydrates: 14.1g
- Dietary Fiber: 6.6g
- Sugars: 4.9g
- Protein: 5.1g
- Sodium: 96mg

TROPICAL GRILLED SCALLOP SALAD

Grilled scallops over a bed of Boston lettuce, accompanied by fresh fruit and drizzled with a tropical-tasting salad dressing that has sweetness and zestiness rolled into one? This is the perfect salad that's dinner-ready in under 15 minutes – need we say more?!

Prep to finish: 13 minutes
Difficulty: Easy
Yield: 2 servings
Serving Size: 1½ cups salad

Ingredients:

- 6 large sea scallops, approximately ¾ pound
- 1 tsp. Emeril's fish rub (or fish rub seasoning of choice)
- Olive oil cooking spray
- (6) ½" thick fresh sliced pineapple
- 2 c. preferred salad greens or a mixture of salad greens
- 2 c. Boston lettuce, torn
- ¼ c. peeled avocado, diced
- 1 tbsp. mango chutney
- 1 tbsp. fresh lime juice
- 2 tsp. extra virgin olive oil

Instructions:

1. To begin, prepare grill for high heat
2. Rinse scallops and pat dry with a paper towel.
3. Sprinkle ¾ tsp. fish rub over scallops. Coat scallops with cooking spray.
4. Transfer scallops to grill and cook about 3 minutes on each side or until they are cooked through.
5. Remove scallops from heat and set aside. Place sliced pineapple on grill, and grill each side for about 2 minutes. Remove pineapple from grill and chop.
6. In a medium-sized mixing bowl, combine salad greens, lettuce, grilled pineapple, and diced avocado. Toss to blend well.
7. Prepare the dressing: cut up the chutney into large pieces. In a small bowl, combine the chutney, lime juice, olive oil, and remaining 1/4 tsp. fish rub.
8. Drizzle dressing over salad mixture and toss to blend well.
9. Place 1½ c. salad on plate. Arrange 3 scallops over salad and serve.

Nutritional info:
- Calories: 247
- Total Fat: 3.6g
- Total Carbohydrates: 20.8g

- Dietary Fiber: 3.4g
- Sugars: 4.8g
- Protein: 30.8g
- Sodium: 559mg

ARUGULA, TURKEY BACON, AND SHRIMP SALAD

Crispy turkey bacon, juicy shrimp, and fresh arugula drizzled in an olive oil and yogurt dressing that packs a ton of flavor into this mouthwatering salad that is perfect for lunch or dinner.

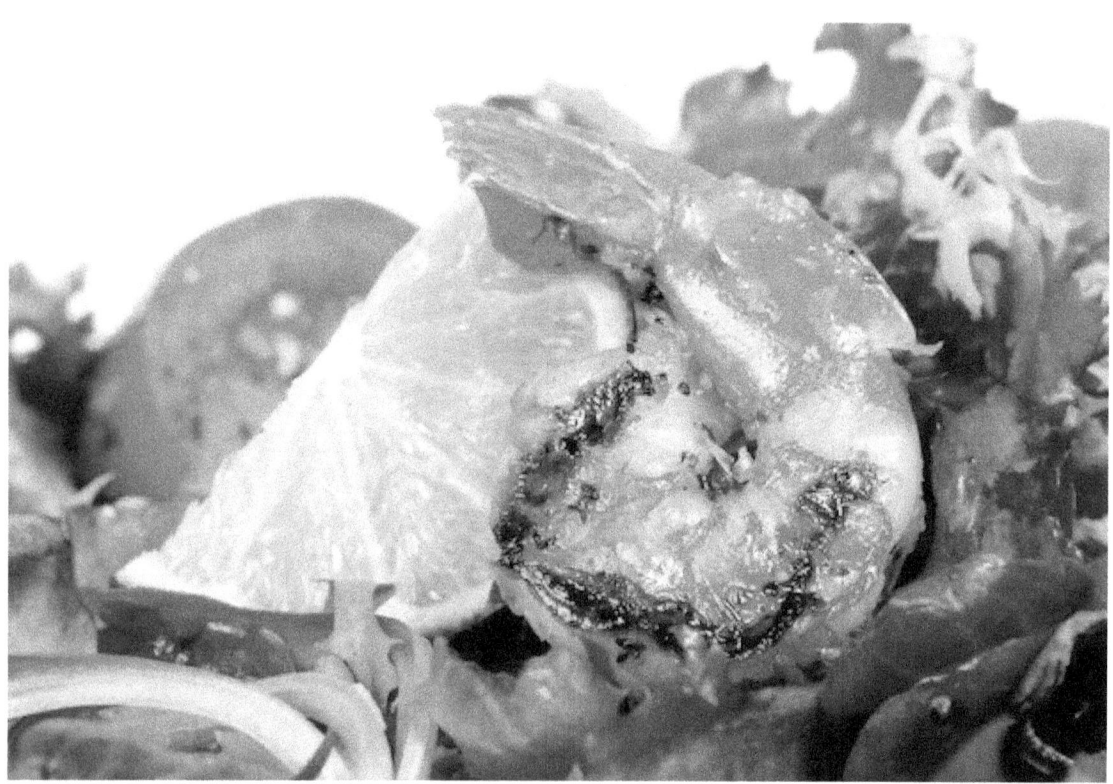

Prep to finish: 30 minutes
Difficulty: Easy
Yield: 4 servings
Serving Size: 2 1/4 cups salad

Ingredients:
- 3 slices turkey bacon
- 12 oz. large shrimp, peeled and deveined
- 5 c. fresh arugula
- 1 c. cherry tomatoes, halved
- 2 tbsp. plain low-fat yogurt (Greek yogurt, if preferred)
- 2 tbsp. balsamic vinegar
- 2 tsp. extra virgin olive oil
- ¼ tsp. fresh ground black pepper
- Sea salt, to taste (optional)

Instructions:

1. Place a large non-stick skillet over medium heat and cook turkey bacon until desired crispiness is reached.
2. Remove bacon from pan and reserve 1 tsp. of the drippings from skillet.
3. Crumble the bacon and set aside.
4. Next, add shrimp to drippings remaining in skillet. Sauté over medium heat for about 5 minutes or until shrimp is cooked through. Remove from heat. With a slotted spoon, transfer shrimp to a large mixing bowl.
5. Add arugula and halved cherry tomatoes to shrimp bowl and toss gently to mix well. Set aside.
6. In a small shallow bowl, prepare dressing by combining yogurt, vinegar, olive oil, pan drippings, and black pepper. Whisk until well blended.
7. Drizzle dressing over shrimp mixture and toss to coat.
8. Transfer 2¼ cups salad to salad plate, top salad with crumbled bacon and serve immediately.

Nutritional info:
- Calories: 166
- Total Fat: 6g
- Total Carbohydrates: 4g
- Dietary Fiber: 1g
- Sugars: 3g
- Protein: 22g
- Sodium: 442mg

ROMAINE-SPINACH SALAD WITH GREEN GODDESS DRIZZLE

Quite the mysterious salad, perfect for those days when a little excitement is in order; the type of day you expect things will be extraordinary and far from simple. This salad is full of antioxidants which will keep you focused, alert, and on the lookout for the unexpected surprises!

Prep to finish: Prep time: 5 minutes
Difficulty: Easy
Yield: 4 servings
Serving Size: 1 salad (see measurements below)

Ingredients:
Green Goddess Drizzle
- ½ c. plain fat-free yogurt (use Greek yogurt, if preferred)
- ¼ c. reduced-fat mayonnaise
- 2 tbsp. fresh flat-leaf parsley, chopped
- 2 tbsp. green onions, chopped
- 1 tbsp. fresh chives, chopped
- 3 tbsp. white wine vinegar
- 2 tsp. anchovy paste
- 1 tsp. fresh tarragon, chopped
- ¼ tsp. fresh ground black pepper
- 1/8 tsp. sea salt
- 1 garlic clove, minced

Salad
- 5 c. fresh romaine lettuce, torn
- 2 c. fresh baby spinach
- 1 c. watercress, trimmed
- 1 ½ c. boneless, skinless chicken breast; fully cooked and chopped
- 2 tomatoes, cut each tomato into 8 wedges
- 2 hard-boiled eggs, each egg sliced or cut into 4 wedges
- ¼ c. avocado, peeled and diced
- ¼ c. crumbled feta cheese (may use crumbled blue cheese, if preferred)

Instructions:
1. Begin by preparing dressing, to do so place first 11 ingredients in the order listed above in a blender or food processor and pulse until smooth. Place in refrigerator to chill.
2. Prepare salad – In a large mixing bowl, combine romaine, baby spinach, and watercress. Toss or use tongs to mix greens thoroughly.
3. On each serving plate, build the salad as follows:
   - Place 2 cups of salad greens on plate.
   - Top salad with 6 tbsp. chopped chicken breast.
   - Arrange 4 tomato wedges on salad.

- Arrange ½ of a sliced egg or 2 egg wedges to each plate.
- Top each salad with 1 ½ tbsp. diced peeled avocado.
- Top each salad with 1 tbsp. crumbled feta or blue cheese.

4. Finally, remove chilled green goddess dressing from fridge and drizzle 1/8 c. dressing over each salad. Serve immediately.

Nutritional info:
- Calories: 249
- Total Fat: 9.8g
- Total Carbohydrates: 14.3g
- Dietary Fiber: 3.8g
- Sugars: 7.9g
- Protein: 23.7g
- Sodium: 637mg